INFECTING THE TREATMENT

INFECTING THE TREATMENT

BEING AN HIV-POSITIVE ANALYST

GILBERT COLE

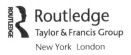

Routledge
Taylor & Francis Group
New York London

First published by 2002 by Analytic Press. Inc.

This edition published 2014 by Routledge
711 Third Avenue, New York, NY 10017
2 Park Square, Milton Park, Abingdon, Oxon OX14 4RN

First issued in hardback 2017

Routledge is an imprint of the Taylor & Francis Group, an informa business

Chapter 1, 2, & 3 are adapted from "The HIV-Positive Analyst: Identifying the Other" published in *Contemporary Psychoanalysis*, Volume 37, issue #1, and appear here by permission.

Typeset in Adobe Garamond by CompuDesign, Charlottesville, VA.

Library of Congress Cataloging-in-Publication Data

Cole, Gilbert W.
    Infecting the treatment : Being an HIV-positive analyst / Gilbert W. Cole.
      p. cm.
    Includes bibliographical references and index.
    ISBN 0-88163-352-6
    1. Cole, Gilbert W.   2. Psychoanalysis—United States.   3. HIV-positive persons—United States. I. Title.
    RC451.4.P79 C65 2002
    616.89'17'092-dc21   2002025351

ISBN 13: 978-0-8816-3352-8 (pbk)
ISBN 13: 978-1-1384-6230-4 (hbk)

To Joe, and the new life he brought to me, and in memory of Mason, for our life before.

CONTENTS

Acknowledgments

Working on a project that involved revealing a great deal of personal detail often frightened me, as if in some way I were tempting fate. This project, of naming very explicitly things that have been stigmatized in the past, seemed often to awaken censorious inner voices telling me that this was not at all a good idea. But when I began to show the work to others, these fears were soothed by responses from many persons. To all these insightful readers, whose empathy and acute critical judgment supported me throughout the writing of this book, I am deeply grateful. Madhu Sarin, Ph.D. read a very early version of some of this material and urged me to develop my ideas. As the work grew, the trenchant editorial suggestions of Patrick Horrigan, Ph.D., Carol Shyer, Ph.D., Jonathan Lebolt, Ph.D., and Elizabeth Minnich, Ph.D. were immensely valuable. Emmanual Kaftal, Ph.D. has been a consistent source of encouragement since long before this project occurred to me. I will always value his guidance and his clinical and intellectual acumen as much as I value his friendship.

Florence Rosiello, Ph.D., Leslie Goldstein, C.S.W., and Roseanne Murphy, C.S.W. offered generous comments on earlier versions of some of this material and calmed much of my anxiety about continuing. Eli Zal, C.S.W., Stephen McNulty, C.S.W., and Bruce Kerner, Psy.D. also read some initial drafts, and their support was valuable to the project. Adrienne Harris, Ph.D. and Muriel Dimen, Ph.D. were other empathic and generous readers of some material. I am also grateful to Mark Blechner, Ph.D., whose acute editorial intelligence and support led to the publication of some of this material in another form. Colin Greer, Ph.D., with an uncanny ability to critique and inspire simultaneously, guided my process writing. Katherine Kuhrs, Ph.D. brought a distinctive point of view in her comments that enriched and clarified the text. At the Analytic Press, the enthusiastic response of Paul E. Stepansky, Ph.D., to the text was a surprise and an inspiration. John Kerr, Ph.D. is an editor whose criticisms were offered with generosity and a collegial spirit. Working on the revisions was a truly enjoyable, creative reexploration. I am also grateful for the care and intelligence of Karen L. Brunson, M.A., Shari Buchwald and Eleanor Kobrin.

Several close friends helped me enormously by simply being available when I needed to express my fears about putting into print not only aspects of my psychic experience and physical health, but also what I believe about how I do clinical work. I will always be grateful for the love and support of Christopher Eldredge, M.A., C.S.W., Charles Rizzuto, C.S.W., and Sheila Ronsen, C.S.W.

I was lucky enough to have been born into a family that is unconditionally supportive and loving. Together with my parents, Jack and Dallas, and my brother Andrew and his wife Kim, I have learned through the years about illness, about loss, and about the importance of never taking anything for granted. I am grateful for their reliable presence during the challenges that have made our intertwined lives so rich.

Finally, I wish to thank my partner, Joe Tribbie, C.S.W., who has had to live with my obsessions and apprehensions for several years of work on this project. He has never been anything but steadfast and loving. I can only hope that he finds me to be so for him.

Preface

THIS CYCLE OF ESSAYS ON THE subject of the HIV seropositivity of the psychoanalyst is the presentation of clinical dilemmas,
fantasies, free associations, and their elaborations that led me to a
more comprehensive understanding of what this status has come to
mean to me. It begins with what at first appears to be a medical
fact, but nothing remains merely a fact for long. We are too full of
life, too creative, and, when pressed by too much anxiety, can become
too obsessive to remain in a world of objective information. We
develop wonderful strategies to organize the realities of our lives. As
psychoanalysts, we involve ourselves in our patients' attempts to
make better strategies when theirs aren't working so well. We all make
stories for ourselves, in very particular styles, in response to the constantly changing expanse of facts and fantasies in which we live.

The medical fact of my HIV seropositivity posed a formidable
series of propositions. If we ask what it means to share information
about a personal medical condition—something about one's substance—in the psychoanalytic encounter, we set in motion a chain
of linkages, amounting to a sort of conjugation of disclosure.
Openness, sharing one's substance, leads to interpenetration, which
leads to contamination. The way that this chain of intersubjective
events rhymes with the action of how I became HIV positive impelled
me to examine the process in greater detail.

If I set out with a fantasy of finding a way to cure myself, in
the end I was convinced that I have no choice but to acknowledge,
even to celebrate, an inevitable vulnerability to infection. As everyone who must adjust to living with an illness learns, the border that

is crossed at the moment of diagnosis has a range of meanings, changing characteristics, and an inconstant topography. There are moments when the salient aspect of carrying a virus is its specificity, whether as a stigma or a marker for being special. At other times, the more prominent experience is the relief that comes with the certainty of ordinary mortality. Hoffman (1998) asks us to consider how our sense of self is compounded of the "dialectic of meaning and mortality" (p. 18). Here I examine the meanings and the difficult relationships I have with my HIV infection, with the tradition and practice of psychoanalysis, and with the complicated relationship between these two significant aspects of my life. It is an attempt to keep a dialogue going, to maintain a dialectical tension, rather than to find a convincing resolution. I offer these observations about problems confronted and created by an HIV-positive analyst in the hope that the specifics of my situation may produce insights and questions that pertain to anyone interested in the psychoanalytic situation.

First, I attempt to delineate aspects of the multiple contexts the problems an HIV-positive psychoanalyst poses and confronts. Psychoanalysis exists in a constantly evolving social and political context. The influences among psychoanalytic ideas, social trends, and political power are mutual and multidirectional. As I consulted the literature on a specific topic (illness in the analyst), I observed these influences in action. And, though it was a particular issue that I followed, I could also clearly read the development of trends of more general theoretical innovation.

I then present a meditation on my own experience of being HIV positive and then several other questions. Arising from the subjective experience of adjusting to a medical fact is the question of the identity that has been constructed from the condition of carrying a latent virus. My aim is to explore the questions of how such an identity is constituted, how it is taken on (or assigned), and what the effects of such a process may be. A practical and clinical context of the effects that a discrete identity rooted in potential illness may have is explored through descriptions of the practice of psychoanalysis and psychoanalytic psychotherapy as an HIV-positive person.

These essays, given life through data gathered through a hybrid method of heuristics, psychoanalysis, and the personal essay, seek to express the subjective experience of phenomena that may have been theorized in part but have not yet been described. These themes include the formation of identity; the imposition of identity; the feeling that one is other (contagious and potentially dangerous); and to have these feelings while practicing as a psychoanalytic therapist. Considering these themes led quickly to the question of disclosure. In this case, it was the disclosure of a medical fact to patients. But I found that the differentiation between a fact and the resonant meanings and feelings connected with that fact, and feelings that I had toward aspects of my relationships with patients, was impossible to maintain. I then come to an exploration of another aspect of the psychoanalytic relationship: as I confronted the question of whether I ought to disclose my serostatus when I met with prospective patients, I had to examine the ethical ground of psychoanalysis that is so easily taken for granted.

The data gathered in conversational interviews with other HIV-positive analysts is then described. These interviews, generally guided by the theme of seropositivity, resemble a fragment of an analytic process, as the subjects were asked to associate freely to such questions as how their condition of seropositivity had impinged on their work; their patients' responses if and when they became aware of their analyst's condition; and whether or not their attitudes about engaging in such a long-term project as psychoanalysis had been affected by their HIV status.

As I began this exploration, I thought that I faced a series of questions concentrically situated one within the other. Instead I found the traces of a series of dissociations. For example, when I set out to locate other HIV-positive psychoanalysts to interview, there was a remarkable lack of response. Clearly no one wished to talk about this subject. Then, interviewing the analysts who were willing to speak with me, I heard what amounted to a shared confession that they had not given their HIV status a lot of thought *with regard to their clinical work*. This omission later related to a similar disavowal of the analyst's vulnerability that is quietly built into both theory and technical recommendations.

Dissociation works again and again: HIV is not so much repressed as set aside. So, too, is sustained thought about illness, vulnerability, and death. There is a paradox here, familiar in psychoanalytic thinking: that the setting aside, a fragmenting, works in the service of holding together. Versions of this unconscious process are manifested in some socially organized practices in which a setting aside of the unacceptable, the irrational, the taboo, or the highly charged is enacted symbolically. In examples ranging from ritual enactments to socially sanctioned quarantine or expulsion, one can observe a process that allows for the splitting off of that which is unmanageable and contaminated. As analysts, we understand particular transference manifestations as functioning in a similar way. This kind of fragmentation and evacuation of sin and badness works to contain the unbearable and unmanageable, protecting us and maintaining a sense of continuity and integration. Fragmentation, a dissociative process, serves an important function in the maintenance of identity.

Pushing a bit further, perhaps the notion of identity itself can be usefully understood as a means of maintaining that process of dissociation in a relational context as an attempt to maintain continuity and integration and in the service of the disposition of power. This relational function often is hidden by dissociative processes, in favor of the naturalizing move of thinking of identity as an essence, permanent and stable. If identity were to be seen as functioning in the service of relational goals rather than as an essence, what type of clinical traction might this imply? What implications might this lead to in thinking through questions evoked by "identity politics"?

The interviews with my colleagues pressed me to rethink writing about psychoanalytic data. Partly because HIV seropositivity continues to be a special case and partly because the psychoanalytic community is so small, I had to find a way to discuss my colleagues' stories with a level of abstraction that protected their anonymity while still allowing for a meaningful specificity. Seeing the material as stories led to the consideration of the meaning carried by the form in which those stories were told. Though we may have certain episodes of the plot in common, my colleagues' narratives unfolded in highly contrasting narrative forms including a romance, an ironic satire, and a gothic horror story. These forms in themselves express salient meanings and carry specific affective charges.

Inspired by my experiences pursuant to disclosing my HIV status, I contend with the notions of disclosure, coming out, and identity. Using a concept borrowed from the discipline of method acting, I conclude with a proposal for thinking through these issues. Functioning as a metaphor for infection, this concept describes what happens in the body of the HIV-positive person and also what happens in any interaction involving two people, especially interactions between parties in the psychoanalytic dyad. The method acting concept also works as a recommendation for a practice of potential value to psychoanalysts, a schema of intersubjectivity that can be experienced by partners working together. In addition, this suggestion carries a highly personal meaning. As I searched for ways to organize and understand the conflicting senses of myself as an HIV-positive analyst, I was surprised at this reconnection to a part of my life that preceded both HIV and my work as a psychoanalyst, when I worked in the theater as an actor. Establishing this link to a past version of myself carries a vitalizing dual awareness of continuity and change. I develop this concept as a metaphor and as a technique in detailing a relational view of the therapeutic situation that maintains the dialectical tension between a one-person and a two-person model of psychoanalytic action.

Technique for the artist, whether in the performing or fine arts, supports and liberates the practitioner. Too often, technique is a source of anxiety for the psychoanalyst. Much of our literature, including some chapters in this volume, are confessions of deviating from standard technique and descriptions of how analysts recovered from their deviations. Perhaps there is a way to rethink a relationship with psychoanalytic technique. To that end, I argue that the method acting concept is useful in thinking about the responsibilities ensuing from a revision of practical recommendations regarding disclosure, anonymity, and abstinence. It is my hope that the presentation of my very specific, limited case experience can set in motion a process of thinking through that will be of value for any clinician interested in the development of psychoanalytic insight and action.

A Communication from the Analyst's Dreamlife

THE NIGHT AFTER I BEGAN to write this introduction, I had the most vivid dream I've had in some time. My recollection of the dream begins in a part of the New York City subway where there are six or eight sets of tracks. I am with two persons I can't identify. We are to be indoctrinated into an underground group of activists who disrupt and demonstrate for the sake of AIDS awareness. Somehow I know that they are all HIV positive and that they've decided to devote all of their energies to a kind of urban terrorism. This group spends a lot of time traveling though subway tunnels on roller-blades, on skateboards, and on carts that remind me of those used by miners. I am struck by the skill of the riders zooming down the tracks, avoiding the electrified third rail. The leader is a young man with long, curly hair who at first looks like the actor Evan Handler. I am afraid, but I am also excited about joining this group.

The scene shifts to a hill or promontory overlooking city hall, and the leader again approaches us. It is the moment of initiation, and he carries a container filled with an iridescent green liquid. He is silent, but I know to open my mouth so that he can dab a bit of the liquid onto my tongue. It is a hallucinogenic, and I begin to have a very pleasant trip. I am aware of being attracted to this strange and apparently wild young man, who now looks like a boy I loved in high school. The moment feels like the point at which I must make an existential choice, one that can never be revoked. I want to make it.

I wake up.

From this dream, I understand that I feel angry. I wonder if there is room in a scholarly piece of writing for my anger, and if my feelings will permit me to work on this project or will be an impediment. By beginning to write this, I am taking another step in coming out, revealing personal information that cannot be taken back. It is a transformational existential moment.

Evan Handler is an actor who had leukemia, who was ill for a long time, and who wrote about his illness in a book and a performance piece that brought him a good deal of attention and professional success. The dream figure he played changed at the end into a brilliant and troubled boy I knew in high school. He eventually left school and spent time in a psychiatric hospital.

Themes of ambition, envy, yearning for love, and confusion about sexual orientation are all present in this dream, along with the predominant story of wishing to undermine all that can be thought of as normal life. It is ironic that, as I write this, nearly 20 years since I probably seroconverted, life with HIV has become normal for me and for my social cohort.

I'm taken aback by this unconscious communication about risk, destructive impulses, and commitment. But it also makes a great deal of emotional sense to have dreamt this dream as I begin to write what I've thought about writing for a long time.

CHAPTER 1

Knots of Meaning

The HIV-Positive Psychoanalyst's Subjectivities

TO APPROACH THE QUESTION—What is the impact of the psychoanalyst's HIV seropositivity on the therapeutic situation?—is to initiate a conversation among converging but disparate discourses. Psychoanalysis, social theory, and politics compete for dominance in this conversation, now supporting, now jostling each other. In this chapter, before focusing on the HIV-positive analyst I wish to identify important aspects of the multiply determined intellectual context out of which that analyst practices. The confrontation and accommodation that characterize the process of this conversation are apparent throughout and are continuous with the development of psychoanalytic literature in general. The capacity of psychoanalytic theory and technique to adapt to social and political change demonstrates the robust flexibility of Freud's original contributions. Through this process, psychoanalysis is nourished as a therapeutic discipline and provides ever more elaborated theoretical tools for social and political theorists' application to work beyond the clinical situation.

In the hundred years since its inception, psychoanalysis has evolved from a relatively unified body of theory and technique to a highly varied, multivocal discipline. Once, psychoanalytic literature scarcely included a description of the psychoanalyst's subjective experience. It was the patient's interior world that was the analyst's only stated focus of attention. Talking about a psychoanalyst from his or her point of view became possible, indeed necessary, through a gradual shift in psychoanalytic thought. The role and function of the analyst's subjective experience has evolved from a countertransference that must be controlled and minimized (Freud, 1915), to an important source of information about the patient's unconscious (Heimann, 1950), to an irreducible part of the therapeutic situation (Renik, 1993). The theoretical orientations that most explicitly discuss the analyst's subjective life are referred to variously as working in a two-person model of treatment, using an interpersonal style, employing a relational perspective, and working intersubjectively. These distinctive theoretical orientations have specific derivations and different emphases, and each overlaps technically and theoretically with the others. This expansion and elaboration of the psychoanalytic discourse is a response to pressures from within the field as well as from social forces, philosophy, and innovative scientific speculation such as complex systems theory. Thinking about the impact of social phenomena on the individual (such as the repercussions of a social stigmatization) was at one time rare in psychoanalytic discourse. The traditional arena of analytic interest was the unconscious fantasy world, often understood to be quite distinct from mundane reality. For the analyst himself to be the object of analytic interest as a person with a stigmatized medical condition is unprecedented.

The HIV-positive person was once thought of, with limited accuracy, as belonging to one or more possibly overlapping groups: gay men, intravenous (IV) drug users, Haitians. One of these groups, gay men, has been an object of psychoanalytic scrutiny since Freud's (1905) "Three Essays on Sexuality." In a sense, the group we now recognize as gay men played a vital role in the constitution of psychoanalytic theory. Homosexual people, "inverts," are his original "test case." Freud begins with a discussion of the "inversion" of sexual instinct toward a member of the same gender. (Although one of Freud's (1920) case studies is of a young lesbian, the psychic experience of lesbians has been relatively neglected in the psychoanalytic literature, often characterizing them as men in women's bodies or viewing lesbian relationships only as regressions to the infant–mother dyad. Recently this lack has begun to be redressed (e.g., O'Connor and Ryan, 1993; Iasenza and Glassgold, 1995; Schwartz, 1998; Magee and Miller, 1999; Schoenberg and Lesser, 1999).

Conversely, psychoanalytic thought has exerted a significant constitutive influence on gay men. Freud (1921) supported the abolition of legislation that discriminated against homosexuals, pointedly arguing against the policy of barring homosexuals from analytic training. Despite his public position, psychoanalysis as a field has notoriously been hostile to gay men and lesbians seeking training, to say nothing of the long history of theoretical literature that pathologizes homosexuality. (For a review of this literature, see Lewes, 1988; and Drescher, 1999.)

The support that Freud publicly offered to homosexual people and the discrimination directed toward this group provided some of the impetus that eventually coalesced into the gay liberation movement of the 1960s. Inspired by the civil rights and feminist movements, gay liberation enabled gay men and lesbians to become a recognizable political group. This political coalescence served as a means of affiliation and as a new source of identification for lesbians and gay men (Duberman, 1994).

HIV has challenged not only medical research and practice but also social policy planning. Research on the virus has yielded knowledge about the human immune system and that class of viruses (retroviruses) to which it belongs. But the social and political history of the first twenty years of acquired immunodeficiency syndrome (AIDS) is full of fear, denial, and stigmatization of the groups in which HIV/AIDS first appeared (Treichler, 1988). Psychoanalysts have provided clinical help to those directly affected by the illness (Blechner, 1997b). Psychoanalysis can also help us to understand why the themes of fear, denial, and stigmatization have been so prominent in its history. Blechner points out that psychoanalysis has benefited by involvement with HIV/AIDS, through the clinical experience gained as analysts care for those who carry the virus. His work with people living with AIDS "taught [him] a level of elasticity beyond what [he] ever thought [he] could work within a psychoanalytic framework" (p. 18).

There is a multidirectional process of interaction in each of the components of the question I wish to put into play. The title I have chosen for this book quite purposefully leads into a complicated knot of subjectivities, theories, and social practices. The word, infecting, is to be understood in at least two ways: as a disclosure of a medical fact about myself, and also as a description of my conviction about a crucial aspect of the psychoanalytic situation. I mean that the intimate involvement of the partners in the consultation room can feel like, at times functions like, a kind of metaphorical mutual infection. The permeability of the boundary between analyst and analysand challenges how we ordinarily think of the ways we transmit the self, or how our identities become known to another.

Before setting out to tease apart some of the components of the complex knot of meanings that the HIV-positive analyst embodies, the intertwining strands must be made explicit. Each strand has its own complex texture. Though an explication of the strands making up this knot must be linear, the relationships among them are not. These are strands of meaning that shimmer and shift rather than remaining constant and binding.

One strand is psychoanalysis, which, as a theory and as a practice, is far from a univocal discipline. So it is important to situate myself among the emerging schools of thought. Developing one's own theory of mind and of practice may have begun with an allegiance to a theoretical orientation or teacher, but rarely does it end there. A lifelong accumulation of clinical experience and reading— of arguing, feeling convinced, and changing one's mind—offer plenty of opportunities for reconsideration and transformation.

Other strands are the social/political/philosophical questions of public identity (including sexual identity) that direct attention to where the personal and the political overlap. For the HIV-positive psychoanalyst who discloses his or her seropositivity, whether in the clinical situation or in life beyond the consulting room, two public identities are explicit: the professional designation and the medical diagnosis. But a further identity is implied because of what we know about the transmission of HIV. That is, whatever ideas others form about how the analyst became infected amount to an identity that is imposed on the analyst. Psychoanalysis, philosophy, and social practice each frame ways of thinking about how an identity is formed and transmitted, making a description of this process particularly complicated.

Hence, for the HIV-positive psychoanalyst, there is a potentially confusing knot of allegiances, identities, and identifications. Each of the strands making up that knot influences the others, and each is informed by individual idiosyncratic subjectivity. And each person's subjectivity has been influenced by the various frames or containers formed through his or her experience prior to HIV seroconversion.

To explicate these strands of meaning, I turn not only to the psychoanalytic literature, but also to the literature that evolved in response to the AIDS pandemic and, briefly, to narratives describing the formation of gay identities. Tracing the mutual interactions among these bodies of literature also reveals a narrative of confrontation and accommodation that I hope leads to an expanded view of psychoanalytic theory and technique. Political organization and changing social practice have forced psychoanalysis into certain confrontations, even while some of these practical phenomena were brought about with the help of psychoanalysis. The accumulated contributions of the individual give voice to the needs that lead to changes of theory and practice. In important ways, the individual is formed and articulated by and through psychoanalytic and sociopolitical ideas. This narrative of my work as an HIV-positive psychoanalyst may be useful as an example through which to examine the process of confrontation, accommodation, and expansion that characterizes the development of the field of psychoanalysis.

A REVIEW OF THE PSYCHOANALYTIC LITERATURE

ON THE PSYCHOANALYST'S ILLNESS AND DISCLOSURE

Schwartz and Silver (1990) use a quote from Freud's (1900) first major work, *The Interpretation of Dreams:* "I knew that I could not go on long with my peculiarly difficult work unless I was in completely sound physical health" (p. 231). Twenty-three years after he wrote this statement, a swelling in his mouth that he had noticed and neglected since 1917 was diagnosed as cancer. From the time of the diagnosis, his closest colleagues helped him to keep this illness a secret. It would be the main cause of his death sixteen years later. Except for private correspondence, Freud maintained his privacy about his condition. And, contrary to his assertion in 1900, he kept a rigorous work schedule for most of the sixteen years after his cancer diagnosis (Gay, 1988).

Freud lived, of course, in a culture that was vastly different from our own. The boundaries around what is considered private and personal seem porous, if they can be said to exist at all, more than a century after Freud's (1900) *Dream Book*. Whereas he advocated an open and honest exposition of tabooed subjects such as sexuality and aggression, his lived experience remained well within the bounds of a bourgeois ethos that required discreet reticence about private matters. It might be argued that Freud's influence has been one factor in the openness that characterizes contemporary popular discourse about subjects once considered too private for public discussion, despite his choice to keep his illness private.

It is noteworthy that few of the analysts who write about their experiences with serious illness mention the precedent Freud set by his silence. Yet consistent in the scant mentions of illness in the analyst are remarks on how little literature there is. It is almost as if Freud's decision has instructed his followers to remain silent as well. Halpert (1982) writes that, as

> some degree of identification with Freud probably exists within every analyst, one wonders whether the image of the 66-year-old man with cancer of the oral cavity, living in pain, struggling on heroically, doing his work through an endless series of surgical procedures until his death at eighty-three, might not form an identificatory model (and perhaps rationalization) for continuing to analyze in the face of pain and death [p. 374].

The heroic ideal is salient, not only with regard to working through one's own suffering, but also to the solitary and isolated quality of the hero's life. Through that isolation, one possible idealized identity for the psychoanalyst is linked to that symbolic figure who is set apart to contain the contamination of others.

The themes emphasized in most of the literature on the analyst's illness are the narcissistic regression that illness causes, the disruption of one's denial of mortality, and the difficulty of maintaining an adequate analytic posture. Many of the contributions to this literature come from analysts working within a classically Freudian technique. So this ideal analytic technique, one that is compromised by the analyst's illness, is the central organizing principle. Within this theoretical point of view a narcissistic regression—theorized by Freud (1915) to be concomitant with any physical illness—and the disruption of one's denial of mortality are viewed as deleterious to the analyst's capacity to function in an optimal way.

The stance Freud advocated for the psychoanalysts is succinctly described in his "technique papers." In "Recommendations to Physicians Practicing Psycho-Analysis" Freud (1912) expresses the hope that his recommendations will spare those who follow him some of the frustrations and mistakes he experienced. He adds that each individual must find his or her own way in the work. The technique, he tells us, is simply described, if difficult to execute: the analyst makes no special effort to concentrate on anything in particular, but maintains an "evenly hovering attention." The analyst, through his evenly hovering attention, works in parallel with the patient, who is directed to freely associate without attempting to censor any of the thoughts passing through the mind. Just how the work is conceptualized is revealed later in this paper, when Freud uses the metaphor of the surgeon, who puts aside all human feelings, including that of sympathy, in order to carry out the operation as skillfully as possible. Still later, Freud states that the analyst "should be opaque to his patients, and, like a mirror, should show them nothing but what is shown to him" (p. 118). Other important aspects of the classically Freudian technical posture include the analyst's *neutrality,* referring to the analyst's stance in relation to the patient's conflicts; the analyst's *anonymity,* referring to the question of the analyst's own disclosures; and the analyst's *abstinence,* referring to the handling of the patient's transference feelings toward the analyst (Hoffer, 1985).

Abend (1982) offers working definitions of *transference* and *countertransference* that apply to much of the literature written by analysts working in a classically Freudian manner. Transference, he writes, refers to

> all the influences of unconscious mental forces . . . the wishes, fears, and defenses of infantile origin, and the complex compromises to which they give rise—on the analysand's relationship to the analyst, as it is perceived, remembered, wished for, and enacted. . . . Our term . . . derives from Freud's initial grasp of the essential feature that they originate in the individual's childhood experiences and relationships. [Countertransference is defined as] a full counterpart of this broad understanding of transference. It includes the impact of the analyst's unconscious mental life—all of the residua of childhood instinctual conflicts—on his or her analytic activity with each patient. . . . [T]his should be thought of as a ubiquitous factor that affects the analyst's work at all times [p. 366].

It must be noted that these definitions of transference and countertransference describe processes that are located in isolated minds, where there is no overlap. There may be, indeed there inevitably are, influences on the other party that result from the transference or countertransference, but according to this understanding of the processes, their origins are clearly differentiated and separate. The intellectual paradigm by which these concepts are organized is strongly influenced by the post-Kantian empiricism that dominated Freud's time and place.

Many of the discussions on the analyst's illness are written from within this paradigm and are expressive of the tension this ideal imposes on the discipline of psychoanalysis. This list includes Chermin, (1976); Abend, (1982, 1986); Dewald, (1982); Halpert, (1982); Silver, (1982); Arlow, (1990); Lasky, (1990, 1992); and Lazar, (1990). The authors detail an ideal analytic stance: that the analyst's work should be analogous to a surgical procedure and that the analyst should be impenetrable, mirrorlike, and thus neutral, anonymous, and abstinent. This ideal stance has elicited many responses throughout the fractious history of psychoanalysis. The contemporary American relational school (e.g., Mitchell, 1988; Aron, 1996; Bromberg, 1998; Hoffman, 1998) is preoccupied with dismantling this model of the isolated mind. In a way, the scant literature on the analyst's illness traces the development of this relational theoretical orientation, one that critiques and deconstructs classical theory, in miniature.

Arlow (1990) offers a gripping description of the moments he fell ill, and advises that what the analyst tells patients (and readers?) about his illness may "express his own defensive need to deny the gravity of his condition" (p. 22). Dewald (1982) discusses the countertransference issues in detail, arguing that the analyst's narcissistic involvement interferes with clinical skills, and that the fantasy of invulnerability to illness and disability leads to the analyst's need to reassert self-esteem and a sense of competence. This need has the potential of leading a recovering analyst to return to work before becoming aware of possible countertransference interference. He also speculates on a fantasy common to analysts, that their own analysis has immunized them against all kinds of illness. Wong (1990) also describes how he decided to give patients factual information about his illness according to an assessment of the quality of the transference and ego strengths of each patient. The more disturbed the patient, the more information was deemed to be required. A patient with a fragile ego structure, who is less able to tolerate ambivalence, needs more information because it is thought that, with this provision, less anxiety is likely to be stimulated by fantasies fueled by unconscious wishes to destroy the analyst. Presumably, such fantasies about the analyst's illness would be ameliorated by factual disclosures by the analyst.

Abend (1982) argues that the post-illness countertransference experience makes it impossible to evaluate objectively whether and what to disclose to patients. He states that he intended not to disclose any information regarding his illness to patients but found it impossible not to, for reasons rooted in countertransference issues. Maintaining the analytic ideal of anonymity is also the most desirable technical stance for Lasky (1990, 1992), but he found that he simply could not live up to it. The strains imposed by the experience of illness proved to be too much. In an attempt to soothe the attacks on himself that he felt he was making, Lasky (1990b) imagined a sympathetic Freud sitting by his side, assuring him that he was still an analyst even though he had deviated from the ideal analytic technique. For all of these analysts there is a clear demarcation between the transference and the countertransference, and the analyst's countertransference is seen as a deleterious factor that must be kept under control.

An article written within the theoretical orientation of British object relations provides a glimpse of shifting attitudes toward aspects of the analyst's private experience, describing their role in the treatment in a different mode. Durban, Lazar, and Ofer (1993) examine the complicated intrapsychic processes pursuant to the analyst's chronic illness. But this is inflected by a definition of the analyst's function and presence that diverges from the heroic ideal of the surgeon who remains transparent and abstinent. In this theoretical view, the analyst functions as a container for unconscious contents, fantasies, wishes, or impulses that are unacceptable to a patient and that must be ejected from the self and projected into the analyst. The analyst must tolerate this accumulation of unacceptable psychic contents until they can be accepted once again by the patient who, through the work of the analysis, has matured sufficiently to reinternalize what was previously intolerable. These authors set out to describe what happens when the analyst is ill, when the container is cracked. They suggest that the crack itself can be a container:

> A confrontation with his own illness may open a gateway for the therapist to a world of contents which bear on the basics of the body and the primitive edges of object relations. This is a world dominated by concrete, pre-symbolic bodily functions, where time is metabolism, internal space is pleasure or pain, fullness or the emptiness of hunger. The readiness to speak and listen to the language of the body is substantially different from succumbing angrily to its constraints; it entails more patience and tolerance on the part of the therapist to his patients' preoccupations with bodily functions and sensations [p. 710].

Thus the analyst's experience of his or her own illness provides a unique access to the most regressed aspects of a patient's experience. These regressed aspects need not pertain to the patient's awareness or experience of the analyst's physical illness. Note that the analyst's experience of regression, due in part to a physical illness, resounds with meaning beyond the illness. In this theoretical approach it is assumed that the analyst's inner experience and the patient's overlap continuously; they interpenetrate. For the analyst working this way, a concern with bodily condition is construed not as a distraction from the patient's experience, but as a greater involvement with it. The question of an objective view of reality has dropped out of consideration, and of central importance is the analyst's understanding of his or her own inner experience as access to the unconscious psychic reality of the patient. The authors do not discuss the question of disclosure, since the patient's inner experience remains the exclusive focus of explicit communication. But the use of the analyst's inner world is remarkably different in this way of working. The separation between isolated minds is breached, and a direct link regarded as a vital method of communication is posited between the unconscious minds of the analytic partners.

A contrasting point of view was expressed in Morrison (1990). Although she did not name it explicitly, her theoretical point of view resonates as intersubjective, rooted in self psychology. This theory and technique favors an empathic connection to patients, as well as close monitoring of the patient's affective state. Self psychology does not posit a technical stance that differs from Freudian technique with regard to disclosures, but, as a developmental arrest model (Mitchell, 1988a), it posits a radically different theory of mind and hence of therapeutic action. The theoretical and technical innovations of an intersubjective approach generally involve the open acknowledgment of the analyst's ongoing, subjective experience. This theory informs Morrison's description of doing clinical work while she was undergoing cancer treatment. She begins with a disclosure of the details of her illness and the emotional meanings it evoked in her as well. She acknowledges that we cannot prevent disruptions in any treatment. We can only consider the "meanings and implications for the treatment of how we handle these situations" (p. 228). She argues that the experience of illness can "enrich and inform the work" (p. 228) and that her capacity for empathy increased. Her description of her mental state is far from the compromised, narcissistic, exhibitionistic state referred to in so much of the literature. Technical decisions are made in different ways: Morrison describes how her disclosures came in response to her patients' associations and questions, rather than according to diagnostic concerns.

The tone of Morrison's papers is remarkable. She begins with a forthright description of exactly what her illness entailed, and includes a generous, affect-laden narration of her subjective experience, a quality that the other papers by women in the 1990 collection of essays (Lazar, 1990, Schwartz, 1990) share in varying degrees. The difference in affective tone between the essays written by men and those by women is striking, a difference that transcends theoretical orientation. Lazar and Schwartz place themselves squarely within a classical Freudian tradition, but they tend to be more open, less preoccupied with their failure to maintain an idealized anonymity, than the male analysts writing on their experiences with illness. I was led to speculate about the potential effects of socialized gender difference on the question of emotional openness as an organizer for this disparity in the tone of the various papers. Echoing a gender difference described in Gilligan (1982), the men seem generally to wrestle with questions of *rules* about disclosing; the women seem far more involved with detailing *nuances* of their *feelings*, as well as those of their patients. Looking to other examples of the expanding literature on the analyst as a person, a body of work dominated by relational/intersubjective points of view, the influence of feminist thought on this branch of psychoanalysis is unmistakable.

ON THE ANALYST'S SUBJECTIVITY, DISCLOSURE, AND COUNTERTRANSFERENCE

This relational theoretical orientation is shared by the authors of essays collected by Gerson (1996). These papers do not discuss illness, but other significant events in the lives of analytic therapists.

Gerson describes her intention in collecting them: "to show how we make clinical use of what we have fashioned from our life encounters as children and adults. Personal struggles with crises or with certain aspects of identity (particularly those of the body-self) sometimes enhance, sometimes limit, but always affect our clinical work" (p. xiii). This implies a divergent point of view both of the role of the analyst and of clinical action. Relational analysts do not assert an objective view of reality or truth, or have a comprehensive view of the meanings of their own, or the patients', behaviors. Self-disclosure is regarded as ongoing and unavoidable, and "analytic anonymity a myth" (p. xiv). Gold (1993) reminds us of the wish for a more than human status: "Although many patients . . . see their therapist as omnipotent and, therefore, problem free, this is . . . *unfortunately* not an accurate perception" (cited in Gerson, p. xvii; Gerson's italics). With that emphasis, Gerson points up the wished-for role that echoes Dewald's (1982) idea that analysts share a fantasy that their personal analyses render them invulnerable to life's inevitable stresses.

In a discussion of a paper entitled "Disclosure: Is it Psycho-analytic?" by Greenberg (1995), Jacobs (1995) remarked that "disclosing information about the personal life of the analyst . . . is quite another, and even more problematic, matter" (p. 240) than the disclosure of the analyst's emotional responses to the patient's material. The clearest expression of the traditional point of view are two essays by Reich (1951, 1960). In this classical view of countertransference, the term is limited to describing the therapist's pathological response to the patient due to the therapist's unresolved conflicts. Disclosure of any aspect of the therapist's experience is vigorously discouraged. Reich argues that any disclosure is a gratification of the patient's wish to witness, and join, the primal scene, defined as a universal infantile fantasy of the parent's sexual union (Moore and Fine, 1990). Thus, disclosures are a disguised seduction, or a response to the seductive pressures coming from the patient. The prohibition of disclosing, which began as the method of preserving the analyst's anonymity, has become implicated in the distinction between abstinence versus gratification of infantile wishes.

Reich's paper came in response to Heimann (1950) and furthered the heated debate inaugurated by that essay, which was the first to describe the use of countertransference as a source of information on the patient's inner world. Written from a Kleinian perspective, the analyst's emotional responses were not reported directly to the patient but provided the basis for interpretations of unconscious material. This approach was detailed and highly refined when Racker (1957) defined the kinds of countertransference (concordant and complementary) and elaborated Heimann's Kleinian point of view with detailed clinical advice. A third contribution to this trend came from Kernberg (1965), who presented the "totalistic" point of view of countertransference, one that encompasses all the analyst's emotional experiences regarding the patient, not merely the responses to the patient's spoken communications. Each of these three papers was highly influential in changing the definition of countertransference to refer to the therapist's total response to the patient. Countertransference, no matter how intense and lasting, has come to be seen as holding valuable information for understanding the patient's psychic experience.

Gradually, too, the question of disclosure of the analyst's emotional response to the patient has widened. For example, Bollas (1987) argues for the analyst's demonstrating a different way of thinking, of *using* his or her own mind, through the disclosure of some emotional responses to the patient. "It is essential to do this because in many patients the free associative process takes place within the analyst, and the clinician must find some way to report his internal processes to link the patient with something that he has lost in himself and enable him to engage more authentically with the free associative process" (p. 205).

And so we see the trajectory that the theorized analytic task has traveled: from an emotional resonance along with the patient's material, to containing aspects of that material that the patient cannot tolerate, to articulating that material for the patient, to demonstrating how the analyst uses his or her own mind as if providing an example for the patient. What were once clearly demarcated regions (two different minds), that led directly to clear technical recommendations regarding anonymity, abstinence, and neutrality, have been rendered less discrete as those boundaries between the analyst's mind and the patient's become increasingly porous.

Jacobs's (1995) cautionary classification of personal data as something quite different directs our attention to the disguises emotional communication can assume. This is one of the arguments expressed by Reich (1951) in support of the analyst's anonymity: that freely disclosing information about one's private life can be quite seductive. The technical recommendations for anonymity express an uneasiness regarding the analyst's capacity to contain his or her own wishes, and the need to protect the patient from them.

Clearly, as revealed by the literature, the border between what is personal information and what is an emotional response can grow less distinct. When pressed to a limit, certain differentiations begin to falter, such as those regarding the *kind* of disclosure, emotional response in contrast to personal information; and the distinctions between disclosure versus anonymity and gratification versus abstinence. The differentiation appears to function as a heuristic device, orienting the analyst in the welter of overlapping pressures. With regard to the subject of the analyst's illness, the literature demonstrates how analysts rewrite this arbitrary distinction between a disclosure of personal data and emotional response, and then hide the overlap. Some information appears for a while to be one thing, then seems to be transformed into something thought (hoped?) to be quite different. We have had to change our way of thinking, from classifying and analyzing entities to participating in a process.

PSYCHOANALYTIC LITERATURE ON HIV/AIDS

It is tempting to claim that AIDS is an emblematic postmodern affliction. A syndrome, rather than a disease, it assumes many forms. It has changed the way many think about illness because it is no one thing, but rather a ceaselessly protean process. AIDS in women has been notoriously underdiagnosed because it manifests so differently than in gay men, in IV drug users, and in children. Even in the body, the virus thought to be associated with AIDS can hide, or it may be obscured when the host's immune system is so robust that it continues to produce millions of T cells despite the damage that HIV causes. In the history of the medical response to HIV/AIDS, there have been so many divergent narratives of the course of the illness that compiling a database with which to guide clinical decisions seemed an impossible task. Before development of the medications that changed HIV/AIDS into a chronic condition, the course of the illness could be strikingly different from case to case, but always with the same ending.

The analytic literature on HIV and AIDS is sparser than that on the analyst's illness. A search of 21 prominent psychoanalytic journals through 1997 yielded only 16 articles that directly confronted questions of working with people living with HIV/AIDS (Stevens and Muskin, 1987; Cohen and Abramowitz, 1990; Sadowy, 1991; Hildebrand, 1992; Blechner, 1993, 1997a; Grosz, 1993; Rosenbaum, 1994; Schaffner, 1994, 1997; Kappraff, 1995; Aronson, 1996; Mayers and Svartberg, 1996; Bauknight and Appelbaum, 1997; Kobayashi, 1997; Olsson, 1997). There are passing references to HIV/AIDS in several articles, often pointing out the syndrome as an example of redrawn boundaries that require rethinking connections between love and death (e.g., Leary, 1994) or as an example of an unusually difficult case to take on (Mayer, 1994).

Schaffner (cited in Blechner, 1997a) tells us that when he revealed to colleagues that he was treating people who were ill with AIDS, one of them asked him why—"What is the use of treating such a patient? You can't cure him anyway!" (p. 63). Schaffner does not speculate as to whether his colleague was referring to the patient's medical condition or to the personality problems assumed to be present in someone who would be likely to have AIDS. This exchange took place early in the epidemic, and it may be hoped that this sentiment is less common nowadays. Fortunately, in response to the gaps in mental health services implied by the attitudes expressed by Schaffner's colleague, an army of therapists arose (many from within the lesbian and gay community) to address the needs of those who were ill. Psychoanalysts, with notable exceptions, were more circumspect in their response, for a variety of reasons.

Blechner (1997a) describes the stigma attached not only to the disease, but also to those who worked with people with the disease at the beginning of the AIDS epidemic. He considers this stigma to stem from psychoanalysis' historical difficulties in addressing the problems of the poor or the socially marginalized, as well as the field's attitude toward gay men. Psychoanalytic literature develops in a sociopolitical context, and psychoanalysts are just as vulnerable as any other human beings to fears associated with stigmatic social identities.

Goffman (1963) points out that the original Greek usage of the term stigma referred "to bodily signs designed to expose something unusual and bad about the moral status of the signifier. The signs were cut or burnt into the body and advertised that the bearer was a slave, a criminal, or a traitor—a blemished person, ritually polluted, to be avoided, especially in public places" (p. 1). Whereas today the term refers to the "disgrace itself rather than to the bodily evidence of it" (p. 2), full-blown AIDS often does mark the body distinctively, advertising what (to many) continues to be a moral status as well as a medical one.

The outbreak of moral censure and panicked calls for extreme measures such as quarantine for groups identified as at risk for contracting AIDS at the beginning of what was then called a crisis has been amply documented (see Treichler, 1988). Understanding the conflicted responses to a medical (and psychological) emergency, it was necessary to face up to the notion that "AIDS is not only a medical crisis on an unparalleled scale, it involves a crisis in representation itself, a crisis over the entire framing of knowledge about the human body and its capacities for sexual pleasure" (Watney, 1988, p. 9). Although eventually it became clear that sexual activity was not the only controversial risk factor for AIDS, sex (particularly between men) continues to be the dominant vector of fear and disapproval, if not for actual spreading of the virus. Thus a medical crisis is imbricated with questions of identities: private, sexual, political.

Goffman's (1963) framework for analysis of different experiences of identity relies on psychoanalytic theory to conceive of "ego identity . . . [as] first of all a subjective, reflexive matter that necessarily must be felt by the individual whose identity is at issue" (p. 106). Distinct from this is "personal identity . . . [which] has to do with the assumption that the individual can be differentiated from all others and that around this means of differentiation a single continuous record of social facts can be attached, entangled, like candy floss, becoming then the sticky substance to which still other biographical facts can be attached" (p. 57). Social identity, broken down further, is defined by Goffman as "the character we impute to the individual . . . seen as an imputation made in potential retrospect—a characterization 'in effect,' a *virtual social identity* . . . [whereas] the category and attributes he could in fact be proved to possess will be called his *actual social identity*" (p. 2). Goffman's analysis presaged the postmodern preoccupation with the effects of power on the articulation and creation of subjectivity, and an aspect of identity that has a strategic function. But that identity must not be regarded as any less authentic because of its utility. In our postmodern culture, where convincing overarching narratives have been undermined, identity construction may be required for strategic reasons: not only for political and ethical motives, but perhaps most important, to foster a feeling of belonging to a community, when communities seem fragmented and transient (Simon, 1996).

Foucault (1973, 1978, 1980) analyzed the effects of power on those upon whom institutions exert their authority, and observed how power tended to create identities that take on private meaning as well as public significance. This process is exemplified by the medical creation, in contrast to the social acknowledgment that long predated its diagnosis, of the homosexual category in 1870, thus providing a source of identification, political organization, psychological explanation, and of course, a means of repressing the deviant (Foucault, 1978). This novel idea, that the sexual object choice of an individual is a meaningful organizer of identity, has proven to be of lasting influence in this age of identity politics. Not only are political beliefs as well as ethnic, economic, and social status seen as meaningful organizers of subgroups, but previously private conditions form lasting and apparently coherent social boundaries. Analogously, HIV/AIDS, and in short order other conditions such as disability (e.g., Linton, 1998), have assumed an influential function as markers of the intersection of private and political/social identities. How it is that social boundaries work to produce an enduring subjectivity links this sociopolitical process to psychoanalysis. This intersection is a location important to psychoanalytic thinking. As Rose (quoted in Watney, 1988) put it, "The question of identity—how it is constituted and maintained— is therefore the central issue through which psychoanalysis enters the political field" (p. 71).

Psychoanalysis defines the process of identity formation as one through which the subject "assimilates an aspect, property, or attribute of the other and is transformed, wholly or partially, after the model the other provides. . . . [I]t is by means of a series of identifications that the personality is constituted and specified" (Laplanche and Pontalis, 1983, p. 205). This is a process that is conducted in two modes: an identification in relation to what is similar in another, and one that is in relation to that which is different in another.

When HIV/AIDS made its first dramatic appearance in the United States, it was in the bodies of homosexual men. By definition, a homosexual man confounds the psychoanalytic description of a masculine identification, as he desires what is like himself, in contrast to the heterosexual man who desires that which is concretely different from himself. More recently, psychoanalytic writers have considered the process of identification to be subtler and to express more variance than the classic equation suggests. Frommer (2000) describes some ways that are not obvious that two men can experience each other as different and the same, implying, of course, that the same may be true of a heterosexual couple.

An excursion into the confusing thicket of the gender/sexual orientation knot is relevant because of the heavy load that the HIV-positive homosexual man's body carries. Miller (1992) defines just how different the construction of the gay man's body is from the straight man's. The "macho straight male body . . . deploys its heft as a *tool* (for work, for its potential and actual intimidation of other, weaker men or women)—as both an armored body and a body wholly given over to utility . . . [whereas the] gym-body of gay male culture . . . displays its muscle primarily as an *image* openly appealing to, and deliberately courting the possibility of being shivered by, someone else's desire" (p. 31). The dichotomous pair comprised of the utilitarian tool opposed to an aesthetic image that is open points up the relationship between the male body and penetration. In the context of infectious diseases, the penetrable body is the most vulnerable. What becomes of desires for penetration then?

Already a source of conflict and shame, the wish to be penetrated becomes inextricably associated with courting death. In an environment marked by the boundaries set by stigma, these conflicts work synergistically with the forced identifications the social surround assigns the bearer of such wishes. Add to this mix the idiosyncratic identifications such a man may have accumulated in the development of his personality and the narrative he has developed to make sense of these identifications, and we have a dizzying array of contending forces doing battle in and on the body of the gay man.

A look at only three vastly divergent examples of contemporary literature explicitly about the establishment of a gay identity reveals markedly different strategies in the battle for self-recognition. Mass (1994) describes how identifications with aggressors became eroticized and thus manageable and integrated. As he, one of the founders of the Gay Men's Health Crisis, witnessed the disaster happening in his most intimate circle, he also confronted his internalized anti-Semitism. To this end, he considered his abiding love of the works of Wagner, a fascination that required him to overlook the racist content of much of that work. The ensuing close examination of how his anti-Semitism was implicated throughout his life, including in his erotic attachments, led to a stronger sense of how deeply his experience had been determined by an anti-Semitic culture, one manifestation of which had been obscured by aesthetics.

Mendelsohn (1999) also examines identity in the context of desire. But for him, there was an erotics of isolation, of remove. He tells us of having "a sense of myself that had been crucial to my identity for as long as I could remember: the part of me that found erotic and intellectual pleasure in the sense that I myself was never wholly in a thing or place or experience, that even as I did and was and lived, there was a part of me I kept in reserve, a space that allowed me a vantage point" (p. 30). Whereas Mass finds strength in integrating a public and political identity, Mendelsohn finds "a new name for myself" (p. 150) in the experience of becoming a parent, in joining a tradition marked as normative.

Boyarin (1997) describes an intellectual quest for identity that entails curing his chronic sense of "inexplicable gender dysphoria" (p. xiii) by reconnecting with a culture where "real men" were "sissies" and reclaiming "the nineteenth century notion of the feminized Jewish male" (p. xiv). He finds in Jewish cultural history a vitalizing antidote to a monolithic construction of masculinity that tends to dominate our contemporary world.

In all of these examples, a reevaluation of the effects of power leads to a rehabilitation of stigmatized identity. The confrontation and revision of aspects of tradition that at first seemed hostile to the individual are transformed into those features whereby the individual recognizes what feels most genuine about the self. "Identity" comes from the Latin adverb *identidem,* which means "repeatedly," so one of identity's meanings is "the same, repeated" (Mendelsohn, 1999, p. 41). The literature on the struggle to find a unique identity reveals the deep paradox obscured by this term.

The social and political presence of a distinctly gay identity provided a focal point for the open expression of homophobia and moral outrage about HIV/AIDS. This response has led to and depended on the creation of an effective set of images associated with the source of fear and disapproval, which served an important boundary-setting function, crucial for containing the anxieties aroused by a mysterious new disease. As Gilman (1988) points out:

> Icons of disease appear to have an existence independent of the reality of any given disease. This 'free-floating' iconography of disease attaches itself to various illnesses (real or imagined) in different societies and at different moments in history. Disease is thus restricted to a specific set of images, thereby forming a visual boundary, a limit to the idea (or fear) of disease. The creation of the image of AIDS must be understood as part of this ongoing attempt to isolate and control disease [p. 88].

Racist as well as homophobic attitudes were implicated in this project of setting an effective boundary of stigma around the disease:

> Heterosexual transmission was labeled by investigators a more "primitive" or "atavistic" stage of the development of AIDS. The pattern of infection in the U.S., where the disease existed only among marginal groups (including blacks), was understood as characterizing a later phase of the disease's history. It was only in "higher" cultures, such as the United States, that the disease was limited to such specific groups as could be immediately and visually identifiable. This creation of a boundary between the infected—labeled and literally seen as different—and the healthy rested on the need to make a clear distinction between the heterosexual, non-IV drug using, white community and those at risk [p. 102–103].

Gilman points out "a powerful secondary effect of the stigma. It clearly defines the boundaries of pollution, limiting the risk to homosexuals (and those other groups now stigmatized) and thus confines heterosexuals' fears about their own vulnerability. The more heterosexual transmission of AIDS becomes a media 'fact,' the greater the need for heterosexuals to retain the image of AIDS as a disease of socially marginal groups" (p. 105).

Because the largest group of people living with AIDS in the first years of the epidemic were middle-class white gay men, many of whom were in psychoanalytic psychotherapy already (often with analysts who were gay), the field had to adapt to this extreme new situation. Describing the modifications in technique that he advises in working with patients who are HIV-positive, Blechner situates his theoretical point of view in the interpersonal tradition of Sullivan, one of the influences on the American relational school. Once again, ideals of objectivity and anonymity are not seen as possible, let alone pertinent. Those theoretical and technical concepts that guide Blechner's (1997b) innovations include "the fundamental question . . . 'what is the patient trying to do?' We need to formulate this question with the patient and then determine whether we can and should help him or her to do it, and if so, how." Also, Blechner states it is important that the analyst have up-to-date medical information on the medical condition and its treatment (p. 13).

Hildebrand (1992) and Grosz (1993) offer descriptions of treatments with two men at different points in the continuum of HIV disease. Both articles are written from a theoretical point of view best described as Kleinian object relations, and both authors remark on their frustration that their patients' homosexuality could not be cured.

Grosz's contribution, a description of how an unconscious fantasy regarding HIV infection is elaborated and expressed in a patient's actions and affective life, is a valuable one. But this is filtered through a theoretical orientation in which contempt is thinly veiled by a purported scientific objectivity. For example, his recounting of the patient's history strongly implies that he regards homosexuality as caused by the familiar recipe of absent father and overinvolvement with mother: his patient described himself, Grosz (1993) says, as "a mama's boy" (p. 965). His own concerns with an origin and explanation of homosexuality affect his analysis of the patient's unconscious fantasy. Grosz interprets what is uncovered in the treatment as meaning that "at a critical level, Mr. A's phantasy of infection is not so much concerned with the origin of his HIV infection, as with the origin of his homosexuality" (p. 971). His patient unconsciously sees his HIV seropositivity "as a result of having been 'poisoned' by his maternal object: that 'poison' is nothing but his *need* for his maternal object" (p. 973). Because homosexuality is understood as a compromise formation defending against unconscious rage at the "maternal object," there is a linkage between needs, poison, and mothers. But it is not at all clear, given Grosz's consistent, perhaps *insistent,* interpretations, beginning in the initial consultation, that the person Mr. A has come to for help is a maternal figure, and that the helplessness Mr. A feels refers more to his early history than to a diagnosis of HIV seropositivity. It is striking that this analyst seems unable to imagine his patient as wishing for a *paternal* object to help him. This point of view is consistent with a traditional psychoanalytic conviction that homosexuality represents either a compromised, defensive relationship with a phallic mother, or an identification with mother such that the homosexual man psychically regards himself as a woman (e.g., Socarides, 1968). There is no room in psychoanalytic theories of this kind for desire that is actually same-sexed. Health is equated with a privileging of difference, and desire for sameness is regressive. Further, sameness and desire are exclusively *genital* sameness and difference (Frommer, 2000).

Grosz (1993) complains that Mr. A was not tested for HIV until the third month of their work together, "some six years after becoming infected" (p. 974), a date we can calculate to be 1988, according to the patient's recollections of having suffered a "flu-like illness." Grosz seems unable to understand what was common knowledge among the gay men whose generation was being decimated at this point in the epidemic: that the only medication available then was AZT, and that its efficacy was highly contested. What Mr. A says, that "it was best not to know . . . a positive result would only make him anxious and disrupt his life . . . there was nothing you could do about a positive test result anyway" (p. 967) was, in 1988, an accurate assessment.

This mutual implication of the search for a cause of homosexuality and the cause of AIDS, as in the case described above, can be interpreted in a different way, as in the work of Isay. His efforts led to the statements issued by the American Psychoanalytic Association in 1991 and 1992 ending their "longstanding but unwritten policy of excluding those who were openly gay or lesbian from training in its institutes" (Isay, 1996, p. 154). His books (1989, 1996) offer examples of psychoanalytic psychotherapy with gay men at various stages of HIV/AIDS illness. He describes the meanings of HIV seropositivity that patients elaborate, particularly the confluence of shame over wishes that are considered feminine, such as the wish to be penetrated by a man. Isay (1996) details the analytic treatments of several men, and includes a description of his own fears of having been infected with HIV. He considers how this fear may have affected his need to give advice to his patients, a departure from his usual analytic posture. He also describes the request of a patient who has been hospitalized to continue his analysis during his stay there. Isay tells us that he moves the hospital bed away from the wall in order to place a chair in his customary position, behind the patient. Though Isay regards this man's wish as indicative of a denial of the strong possibility of his death, it was also clear that the patient was committed to an analytic, exploratory treatment. In time, Isay tells us the treatment was useful in addressing the issues of AIDS and death, as well as the characterological problems that led this patient to analysis. It is remarkable that in these cases, there seems not to be a preoccupation with a *cause* of homosexuality. These patients know that they are working with an openly gay analyst. They are able to direct their attention to other matters, as their analyst is not at all interested in *changing* their sexual orientation.

Beyond a strictly psychoanalytic point of view, there are many significant contributions to psychological literature on HIV/AIDS. Goldman's (1989) contribution emphasizes the strains of "bearing the unbearable" (p. 263), not only on those affected by the illness directly, but also on those psychotherapists and physicians who work with them. Goldman's article is notable in that he includes the remarks of another psychologist who is diagnosed with AIDS, clearly stating that those called upon to care for those affected by HIV/AIDS are sometimes infected themselves. Goldman also movingly describes the funeral of one of his own patients, who had requested an informal memorial at which friends and family would speak. Noting the difficulty the group had in beginning, Goldman relates how he spoke first, "sharing knowledge that a psychotherapist is almost never justified in doing during the usual practice of our profession; these are not usual times" (p. 273–274). The readiness of the psychotherapist to adapt to challenges, at times being willing to forego the comforts of standard technique, is a crucial point that he addresses.

Because the psychotherapeutic literature outside of psychoanalysis originates in a point of view where concerns with transference, countertransference, neutrality, and abstinence are little emphasized, if at all, I will cite only three other contributors. Schwartzberg (1993) discusses the idiosyncratic and often conflicting meanings that HIV/AIDS has for each individual who is infected. He describes a sense of belonging in many gay men who find that they are HIV positive. Here he points to the way that a diagnosis can become a basis for identification: a different, alarming, way of recognizing oneself. This same intimation of belonging to a new subgroup is also isolating. When a friend tests negative, those who are HIV positive find it difficult to be as celebratory as they feel they ought to be. Schwartzberg (1994) posits four modes of making meaning among HIV-positive people: high meaning, defensive meaning, shattered meaning, and irrelevant meaning. Odets (1995) has pointed to the inverse of the dynamic by which HIV-positive people feel a new sense of belonging, in his description of HIV-negative men who feel invisible, without recognition, alone. Working without discrimination on those who were infected and not infected, he found that HIV quickly took on the power to create meaningful identities.

One psychotherapist who has courageously written about his own condition of HIV seropositivity and the difficulties of working with others who are HIV positive and have AIDS, is Shernoff (1991, 1996). In his writing, he emphasizes difficulties with maintaining a sufficiently empathic stance while feeling overwhelmed, angry, and frightened that what he observes happening to his patients will eventually happen to him. He describes a paradoxical sense that it is his condition of being HIV-positive that enables him to have a special empathy for his patients, while being on guard not to allow himself to "drift off into thoughts about my own condition" (1991, p. 233). He works to find a way to "distance myself from the difficult feelings, without distancing myself from the patient who is discussing and eliciting the feelings" (1991, p. 233).

Note the need to maintain enough distance from the patient (to avoid interpenetration) in order *not* to become preoccupied with his own condition. A therapist working within a psychoanalytic point of view, and particularly a relational one, might permit exactly that to occur, in order to understand something about the ongoing quality of the relationship that is unfolding between analyst and patient.

All the literature concerning illness—whether in the analyst or not, whether it is HIV/AIDS or not—contributes to a narrative that tells an implicit story of shifting, porous boundaries. In this way, illness (perhaps HIV/AIDS in particular) seems to exert an effect on psychoanalytic theory and practice that echoes the development of some crucial ideas of the contemporary American relational school of psychoanalytic thinking. As Schwartz (1990) asserts in his introduction, it is the accumulation of particular stories of analysis that create the "rich source of subtle data on the very essence of what makes a relationship psychoanalytic" (p. 3). I go further, and suggest that even the stories told from within a classically Freudian point of view lead us toward an unavoidable interpenetration, the dynamism of which makes psychoanalysis relational.

PSYCHOANALYSIS AS RESEARCH METHOD: PROBLEMS OF INTENTION AND FORM

The therapeutic goal of psychoanalysis is to understand and modify subjective experience so that the subject gains more freedom in the capacity to love, to work, and to play. Because the first step in helping a patient to change is understanding his or her subjective experience in as much detail as possible, research into subjective experience is necessarily a part of the therapeutic process. Freud succinctly described the psychoanalytic method in terms of working with dreams in *Interpretation of Dreams* (1900). His method, generalizable to material other than dreams, consists of breaking down the dream (memory, image, or idea) into its smallest components and allowing the mind freely to associate to each part. As the links and discontinuities between associations are traced, an underlying narrative emerges. Through this process a fantasy, or narrative, that has remained beyond awareness but has infused the object of study becomes available to consciousness.

Breuer and Freud report that it was Anna O, famously regarded as the first truly psychoanalytic patient, who suggested the basic technique. Breuer tells us that "It turned out to be quite impracticable to shorten the work by trying to elicit in her memory straight away the first provoking cause of her symptoms" (Breuer and Freud, 1895, p. 35). Perhaps it was because Anna told him to stop asking questions and simply listen to her that he realized that he had to keep quiet and allow her to do in her own way what she called "chimney sweeping" (p. 30), that is, she free associated. The way Breuer learned Anna could work with him became the basic psychoanalytic rule: that the patient must be permitted to say whatever comes to mind, without censorship or comment from the analyst. This rule remains central to any psychoanalytic practice, whatever innovative contemporary theory informs it.

But it is important to keep in mind the differences between a therapeutic discipline and a research methodology. Psychoanalytic claims to having uncovered basic research data on psychic functioning have been criticized on such issues as generalizing from very small samples the ubiquity of the oedipus complex or penis envy in women. Critics accuse psychoanalysts of being guided by an ideology that means they already know what they are looking for, rendering any conclusions purporting to be valid research data as questionable at best (Grunbaum, 1984). It is convincingly argued that psychoanalysis simply cannot conform to empirical research designs, and some argue that psychoanalysts ought to give up trying to do so.

Edelson (1984) describes the lengths to which psychoanalytic researchers have gone in order to comply with the empirical paradigm. One approach has been the single-subject case study, where an accumulation of cases of similar profile might provide a sampling of statistical significance. But, because these studies are usually composed of extremely small samplings, where random samples are impossible to gather, there is considerable and perhaps irrefutable skepticism on the question of generalizability of data presented in this way.

Contemporary psychoanalysts have refined and developed an intersubjective theory that remains more attuned to the particularities of the patient's experience, moving further away from a theoretical knowingness that has made the field vulnerable to such criticism. In a way, these innovations have moved psychoanalysis closer to qualitative investigations such as heuristic, hermeneutic, and phenomenological research methods. Contemporary psychoanalysts explicitly invoke the hermeneutic discipline in theoretical descriptions of clinical technique, and in many ways the research methods based in these philosophically derived points of view overlap significantly with psychoanalytic theory of technique.

Consider one example of a psychological research paradigm inspired by heuristics. Moustakas (1990) describes the goal of his approach as attempting to recreate a lived experience *from the point of view of the subject.* This is a succinct expression of a goal of one school of psychoanalytic thought, Kohut's (1971, 1984) self psychology and the intersubjective group that has grown from it, which has been extremely influential for many contemporary clinicians. Because of this consonance, a heuristic method seems to be the most appropriate paradigm with which to begin. The data gathered take the form of my subjective writing, transcripts of analytic sessions with my own patients, and tape recordings of interviews with other HIV-positive analysts. These data are worked over and organized in such a way as to describe the experience of each HIV-positive analyst, and, in the cases of my patients, their impressions of the effect my disclosure has had on our ongoing work together. After a period of "immersion and incubation" (Moustakas, 1990, p. 28), emergent insights as to the constituents of the subject's experience gradually became available to conscious awareness, and so permit a fuller explication of, and speculative fantasies about, the experience of being an HIV-positive analyst.

However, there are important differences between a heuristic research method as conceptualized by Moustakas and the psychoanalytic research I wish to describe. Moustakas's goal is to locate and distill subjective reports down to an essence. What is of interest to me in this exploration, as a researcher and as a psychoanalyst, is to locate and amplify what is particular and discontinuous. Undoubtedly, psychoanalysis and heuristic research overlap in terms of concepts that animate both disciplines: for example, this study required long and repeated periods of reflection on the meanings associated with being HIV positive that I've constructed, and on the ways patients of mine and other analysts construct their own meanings about this. But I hold all the products of this work differently—not as helping to define an essence, but as revealing a process that occurs in a relational context that is contingent, multiply determined, and shifting.

The theory of human subjectivity that is implicit in the heuristic research defined by Moustakas is one of abiding wholeness, culminating in the expression of a selfhood that achieves its full flowering under optimal conditions. This narrative of a development of self and identity has a heroic arc. It is enormously appealing for a variety of reasons, and analogies to natural phenomena (the growth and development of physical bodies, the blossoming of flowers, the ripening of fruit) bolster a sense of the naturalness of this narrative. Of course, this need not be a trend inherent in any research paradigm inspired by a heuristic method.

Psychoanalysis, with its interest in the exception, holds a certain appeal to critics, like myself, of the heroic narrative of self-development. It offers a way of locating, amplifying, and articulating the schisms, the fragmentations, the discontinuities that reveal the narrative of a natural flowering of selfhood to be a subjectively constructed wish, rather than an empirically demonstrable condition of human experience.

There is a further problem confronting any psychoanalytic researcher, that of the relationship between psychoanalysis and research into human experience. However much we'd like this to be a transparent relationship, we must face the fact that it cannot be. First, because a psychoanalyst's relationship to subjects of research may also be that of therapist to patient (and so, quite intimate), the shift from a therapeutic role to an observational one risks effecting changes in that relationship. The way in which those changes are worked through adds a burden to the therapeutic task. Second, there is the question of the form in which we present our data. From the beginning of psychoanalysis, the necessity to demonstrate the legitimacy and authority of psychoanalytic claims has forced analytic therapists to confront the problem of presenting material from therapy sessions. This presents certain limitations and challenges the capacity of psychoanalytic writers to establish a narrative authority in a situation in which they are intimately involved, while protecting the most intimate and privileged of material.

It might even be said that the solution to the problems of presenting convincing psychoanalytic research data has yielded a distinct literary genre with its own particular voice: the case study of the unconscious. Freud's (1909) stories of the "Rat Man" and the "Wolf Man" (1918) have often been compared to detective stories, but the mystery and the crime take place in terrain quite different from that in the tales of Poe, for example, however psychologically prescient these are. Freud's expansive imaginative license strains against traditional literary classification. Over time, the psychoanalytic literary genre has expanded, taking on a variety of other qualities. Examples might be described as the *confession*, in which the analyst describes a departure from classical technique; the *meditation*, in which the analyst engages in a wide-ranging speculation based on his or her private experience; and the *koan*, in which the analyst presents a conundrum or paradox and then explains how this is useful. Freud's less widely known, highly speculative essays find him involved in conversations with himself, trying to think through problems that seem to defy logical explanation, such as "The Uncanny" (Freud, 1919).

As I consider where in psychoanalytic literature this contribution might be situated, I turn to the tradition of the personal essay. Lopate (1995) argues that

> the essay form as a whole has long been associated with an experimental method. . . . To essay is to attempt, to test, to make a run at something without knowing whether you are going to succeed. . . . There is something heroic in the essayist's gesture of striking out toward the unknown, not only without a map, but without certainty that there is anything worthy to be found. One would like to think that the personal essay represents a kind of basic research on the self, in ways that are allied with science and philosophy [p. xiii].

Crapanzano (1992), in a similar vein, asserts, "The essay enjoys a freedom, a tentativeness, and a speculative possibility that do not exist in the insistent paper or the determined article. Behind them lie an epistemology of certitude, a politics of final authority, and a bracketing of the ethical" (p. 1). Further, the essay "gives us the possibility of expressing some of the speculative fantasies that are conventionally eliminated in the sacrificing rigor of thought, a play, an irony, a critical awareness that is for me at the heart of the human sciences" (p. 2).

This research endeavor is continuous with the psychoanalytic tradition that Freud inaugurated: a conversation with myself in the form of personal essay, which Lopate terms basic research on the self, and located, as Crapanzano asserts, at the heart of the human sciences.

CHAPTER 2

THE HIV-POSITIVE ANALYST

An Anomalous Identity

IT HAS JUST HAPPENED AGAIN. Earlier this week, I had blood drawn for a T cell test, in order to decide whether I should begin to take the recently available protease inhibitors. In the 10 years that I have had quarterly blood tests, the same sequence of psychic events has occurred. I begin by asserting once again how ridiculous it is to allow numbers that measure a component of my blood to determine how I experience myself. Then the familiar fantasy begins, that suddenly this dreadful, decade-long mistake will be over. In my fantasy, I telephone the doctor's office for the result of the blood test and an alarmed and excited nurse tells me that the reading is well within the normal range and that in fact there has been a terrible mistake: I am not HIV positive at all. Then comes the bargaining period, in which I attempt to end my reliance on this kind of denial by assessing the realistic aspects of the situation. I take into consideration all the clinical facts of my physical state, as well as the significant progress in treating the virus. And then, after firmly telling myself to calm down, I call the doctor's office and receive the news.

I tested positive for HIV before I began my psychoanalytic training but after beginning analysis, and after deciding to become an analyst. The chance of testing positive did not seem unrealistic even as I was deciding to become an analyst, and so a cognitive dissonance emerged that had to be negotiated: did it make sense to begin a lengthy training period in order to engage in a protracted, intimate process with other people while I harbored a potentially devastating virus in my body? The intimation that such a negotiation was necessary can be regarded as a prescient sign of the potential constructions of myself that seemed latent along with the effects of the virus. Perhaps it is an indication of the wish to dissociate any of the inevitable new constructions that I considered only for a brief moment what it would be like to tell anyone with whom I would be involved professionally about my serostatus. I believed I could keep that more or less a secret in my work as an analyst. That was long enough ago that the prognosis for anyone who had tested positive for HIV was at best 10 to 12 years of life. I exercised a crucial and healthy denial in order to complete my training. Then denial stopped being crucial and healthy.

In March of 1996, the William Alanson White Institute presented the first analytic conference devoted to HIV and AIDS. "HIV and Psychoanalysis" was, to my knowledge, the first organized, explicit response to HIV from the psychoanalytic community, and it occurred 11 years after the virus was isolated. Even though I felt that this conference was long overdue, I was enthusiastic about attending. The individuals who had organized the event were dedicated pioneers in the analytic field. But as I read the program of conference events, I was struck by the fact that nowhere was there a hint of the existence of the HIV-positive analyst, as if such a creature did not exist. Yet there I sat, my presence marking this absence of reference. I felt very alone in an auditorium full of colleagues. Was this a moment when I should "out" myself, if for no other reason than to work against a dreadful feeling of invisibility?

When I asked the panel in the morning session about this absence, the responses were important. We were told that HIV-positive analysts do, in fact, exist but that support was sought in the interest of keeping their status a secret so that they could keep on working. Bert Schaffner told us about facilitating a group for HIV-positive physicians, including analysts, in which keeping the secret of HIV positivity so as to maintain a practice was a central concern. This group had been formed early in the history of the AIDS phenomenon, so this was completely logical. In his response to my question, Mark Blechner pointed out that the analyst's privacy, particularly when he or she is confronting so stigmatized a condition, must be protected. In 1996, privacy may still have been of paramount importance. But, in the 21st century, is keeping HIV-seropositivity secret still the only option for an analyst?

As I prepared to raise my question, I experienced a nauseating wave of anxiety. To point out the absence of HIV-positive analysts felt tantamount to identifying myself as one of that group. Although everyone, when pressed, would admit that such therapists must exist, a creeping notion, rooted in the ideal of the analyst's neutrality, had taken over the analytic landscape like kudzu, leafing out into a fantasy of the analyst's naiveté and inviolability. As far as I knew then, few mental health professionals, and fewer analysts, had made their status a matter of record. Why was I about to actively reconstruct myself in this way? "What does it mean *now*, apart from what has it meant in the past, to assert one's seropositivity?" I wondered. As I framed my question, I wondered, too, what consequences there might be to my disclosure. I had already identified myself as a therapist who worked with people affected by HIV. At times throughout the last several years, my practice has been made up predominantly of people coping with one phase or another of the spectrum of HIV infection and AIDS. Were it to be generally known that I am HIV positive, would my referrals become limited exclusively to those who are HIV positive or living with AIDS? Would I no longer see any HIV-negative patients, heterosexual or homosexual? Would all my referral sources dry up as people feared referring patients to an analyst who might sicken and die prematurely?

Why does an analyst reveal anything personal to a patient? Is there justification for any sort of revelation as a viable course of action? Concerns with mutuality and authenticity in the analytic situation have become prominent in contemporary literature (e.g., Aron, 1996; Renik, 1995b), but authenticity is hardly predicated on revealing aspects of one's personal (let alone medical) situation. A public assertion of a status that has remained for the most part invisible within the analytic community is not to be equated with the establishment of an authentic presence in clinical work. But the question that is raised concerning the articulation of identity seems particularly pressing in the circumstances in which I have found myself.

Since the 1960s, with the feminist movement's fervent assertion that the realm of the personal and private cannot be so neatly sequestered from the political and public, the ideal of the self-conscious articulation of identity has been a valued signifier. In our lives now, the state encroaches in increasingly menacing ways on what is easily taken for granted as the private. Matters of choice in abortion, privacy of sexual acts between consenting adults, and the autonomy of mental health professionals to treat their patients are all areas that are already under the scrutiny of some representative body of the state or are at risk of becoming so. In a letter to the editor of the *New York Times* on August 26, 1997, a psychiatrist advocated that health care professionals who were HIV positive and symptomatic or who had AIDS be registered in order to guard against risks posed by clinicians who had become demented because of the virus. This rather alarming suggestion carries many meanings, not least the risks inherent in identifying oneself as seropositive to those who have grave apprehensions about what that means.

As an HIV-positive analyst, I have found it necessary to articulate responsibilities to myself about disclosure. My concern with maintaining a stance that felt false with certain patients was the impetus for my considering the question. I had for several years practiced without informing any patient of my serostatus. Then, when my work became predominantly with HIV-positive patients, the question of disclosure became crucial. Some patients asserted that they wished to work only with an HIV-positive therapist. Does the encounter with a potentially life-threatening illness lead necessarily to a change in the analytic stance in order to gratify such a wish? The body of theory that would assert a negative reply to this question directs our attention to the patient's psychic reality; to fantasy, wishes, conflicts; and to the transference. But is there a way to consider this question without limiting our options to disclosure versus anonymity? Are we forced into a position that somehow pits the patient's needs against those of the analyst? I believe that the tension emerging from the effort to include both a one-person and a two-person perspective on the analytic encounter generates more possibilities and harder decisions for the analyst. For example, maintaining relative anonymity, can we assert confidently that the patient of an ill analyst does not know that something is wrong before the analyst confides it? Perhaps the HIV-positive analyst has a responsibility to reveal this fact to all patients, in the event that his or her health does begin to deteriorate.

The condition of being HIV positive is, in important ways, unlike other physical conditions that may impinge on the analytic dyad. One significant difference is that the state of seropositivity is invisible. While the HIV-positive individual is not sick, however, and his or her physical appearance is not altered in any way, there may be a pervasive sense of potential destructive or dangerous power. It is as if he or she is transformed on a cellular level by seroconversion. One HIV-positive patient told me that he thought of his blood as radioactive. It possessed a charge, doubling the positive trait we all share, the fact of having blood in the first place. He was aware that he looked fine, but he could not escape a sense of the imminent danger he posed to others simply by being. In his fantasy, the threat of infection occurred not through contact with bodily fluids but through some other, seemingly osmotic process: he *was*, therefore he was infectious. His doubly positive existence meant that he was always already interacting, penetrating, and infecting, a danger to others.

This man's fantasies were determined by his idiosyncratic organizing principles, as well as by the fantasies of contagion (which seem to be contagious, too) that circulate through the culture in which we live. It is significant that a magazine originating in one sector of the HIV-positive community is called *Diseased Pariah News*. Recall the extraordinary notions about AIDS when the syndrome first appeared: that it was *caused* by the introduction of semen into the rectum by homosexual activity; that it was a plot hatched by some government agency to wipe out gay men, or African-American people. Before the virus was isolated, the disease was understood as a punishment for the transgressions of those suffering from it, marked as they were as part of a devalued and hated group. Eventually, when certain others who had AIDS could no longer be ignored, such as hemophiliacs or children of the sexual partners of IV drug users, the term innocent victim was used. As Sontag (1988) points out, the term *innocent* simultaneously evokes its partner, *guilty*. In the metaphoric construction of a disease like AIDS, there is no such thing as innocence. In one infamous incident, children who had seroconverted as a result of transfusions were forced to move away from the town in which they'd always lived; their house was burned down. Even innocent victims have not been sheltered from the perception of guilt, contagion, sin, and danger. An instant culture of shame and disgust formed around the illness, as it became a lightning rod for all that was split off and denied about forbidden wishes and fears.

A nodal point in this discourse is the problem presented by the man who desires to be penetrated by another man. Although recent data alerts us to the fact that oral sex presents a greater risk of transmission of HIV than previously believed, it is thought that anal intercourse is the sexual behavior that puts an individual at greatest risk for exposure to the virus. What greater flash point can there be for a heterosexist culture? The fact is that the avowal of such desires—one that may be implicit in the public assertion of one's homosexuality (and almost certainly is in the gay man's admission of HIV seropositivity)—marks the man making these statements as guilty of transgressing the salient boundaries of our culture's construction of masculinity. Conservative Boston talk-show host David Brudnoy (1997), who has publicly disclosed his HIV-positivity and homosexuality, emphasizes his assertion that he has never engaged in anal sex. This claim highlights the charged ambivalence that surrounds the notion of a man's desire to be penetrated. For corroboration, one need only point to the demands that HIV-positive people be quarantined, despite the relative difficulty of transmitting the virus (unlike tuberculosis, for example). It is not difficult to hear the echoes of my patient's private, unreasonable fears of his infectious potential in the world outside. The fantasy of a fundamental, frightening transformation is held and expressed by both the individual and the social surround. We note too how the discourse quickly devolves into the stark and simpler world of paired opposites: positive–negative, normal–perverse, silence–disclosure, healthy–diseased.

And so, the question: why name myself in this way when I could easily remain invisible? Shame, fear, and the seductive power of fantasy all argue for silence. Indeed, one of my recurring fantasies has always been that my health would stay stable long enough for me to benefit from medical progress in treating HIV, that I would remain unmarked and nameless until the problem of naming myself went away. In a sense, I relied on reversing the coming-out process. As some researchers and doctors have, for the first time, begun talking about curing or maintaining HIV infection like a chronic disease, part of my fantasy may become operable. It may be that I will not progress to AIDS. But the problem of naming myself does not simply go away. Because the HIV-positive person usually bears no outward sign of difference, he lives in the space between being sick and well. The experience of existence in this space requires a negotiation of a new narrative of self. But the stress of existing between these poles is difficult to withstand. There is tremendous pressure forcing the HIV-positive person into the category of Other. One of the remarks my doctor made to me at the time of my positive HIV test was that I was "*joining* a very large club." He reminded me that in New York, there is a larger percentage of HIV-positive people than the total population of some small cities. This is just one example of the manner in which the patient is named and set apart as Other against his volition. What felt more accurate was that I had been *assigned* to a new social group. Whether that group ought to be called a club, and whether and how a person joins it, were questions that remained for me to explore.

In the first decade after the discovery of AIDS, it was noted that HIV indeed constituted a category and so was a means to dispose of despised groups. As Foucault (1973) argued, one function of medical pathology has been the construction of illness as a means of social control. He showed us how the medical gaze constructs the clinical object in order to separate it from the rest of society. There was a time in the history of medicine when the sick were treated in the home and the community. Progress in medical knowledge and expertise led to the creation of the hospital, serving multiple functions. Not only was infection contained, but the fearful sight of the diseased and insane was removed from daily life. When what is feared becomes stigmatized, this process demonstrates how humans require reviled groups in order to recognize themselves. If not HIV, then another marker for the Other—who bears what cannot be tolerated or named, but without whom we are not complete—would be constituted by and for the gaze of the defining subject. The endless and impossible struggle to obliterate what cannot be tolerated signifies our terrible struggle to recognize what we dread but cannot escape desiring.

So what would it mean to embrace this designation of Other? To name oneself as part of what is dreaded, disowned, and yet impossible to live without is both a social and a private act that is inherently revolutionary. Each of us who claims the difference that is represented by our seropositivity volunteers our body as a site for recognition of the Other, an act that can be rendered more potent if it is possible to straddle the categories of Self and Other. And here we note a repeated reworking of the ambivalence of the first object relationship. Lacan has argued that Desire is the desire of the Other, and that Other is the self that we struggle to recognize and not to recognize. This constructed image of ourselves occurs at what Lacan (1977) termed the mirror stage. Here is the moment when the infant recognizes that the image in the mirror is itself; that the infant is in the mirror. This is a triumph for the child. "The mirror image is a minimal paraphrase of the nascent ego" (Bowie, 1991, p. 22). But this image is a derisory illusion: a fantasy that there is an objective, substantial entity we can point to as a self. Captivated by the spatial relationship between the reflected image and the real body, the infant is indeed captured by this decoy of a self. At this moment, the person is alienated from the self in process, or a dynamic becomingness. Such becoming cannot occupy a discrete location. The spatial relationship predicated by the illusion of the self in a discrete location initiates a conception of the self as divisible and divided. When the self is recognized by this sighting "out there," an infinite regression of images, as seen between two facing mirrors, instantly comes into view. Among the reflections that bounce down that infinite regress are fantasies about the other.

The phenomenon of AIDS forms an intersection with masculine fantasies concerning interiority that carry particular salience in the question of the construction of identity. Anxieties about the other that is inside have long been a masculine preoccupation. Perhaps this is an expression of the male's envy of the generative power of women. Recall the Greek myth of the origin of the Olympic gods. Cronos, having been told that a child of his would overpower him, demanded that his wife give him each of their children as she gave birth, and he swallowed them. She hid her last child, Zeus, and gave Cronos a stone wrapped in swaddling instead. She then gave him an emetic potion, and Cronos vomited up Zeus's five siblings, who, along with their brother, rose up against their father, killed him, and became the rulers of Olympus (Aldington and Ames, 1959). The price the male must pay for containing life within is his destruction.

The Greeks elaborated on the fantasy of the male's generative capacity in other ways: for example, the birth of Athena, whose mother, Metis, transformed herself into a fly that Zeus swallowed. Inside the god, Metis fashioned a helmet and breastplate and gave birth to their daughter, who sprang full grown from Zeus's head (which had been split open by Hephaestus). Another myth involves the gestation of a child that has been sewn up in the flesh of the god's inner thigh. Along with the expression of male envy of women's capacity to bear children is anxiety about one's interior. As if to deny fears of fragility, heads are split open to no disastrous effect. The body that can harbor new life also harbors its own destruction, as in the Cronos myth, or it can fragment and reconstitute. Fantasies of merging self and Other overlap here with fears about what is inside of the self, unformulated and unknowable. What can the body contain? Can the Other be contained in the self? Can the self be contained once again in blissful reunion with mother?

But the body can so easily become a traitor. The spatial relationship of Lacan's mirror stage, where the state of being captivated easily slips into decapitation, finds representation in fantasies about fragmentation of the body. The paintings of Hieronymus Bosch are perhaps the best exemplification of this unconscious fantasy in which the fragmenting body, a sadistically mutilated version of the self that must be disavowed, is deeded to the other in revulsion (Bowie, 1991). The fragmented body is the site of the struggle to avoid recognition, and the persistence of the fantasy attests to the unflagging battles for the yearned-for recognition.

At the same time that some epidemiologists suspect that the AIDS virus was silently spreading itself through urban-American gay society, contemporary popular culture elaborated the fantasy of the meanings of the voluntary siting of the body as a battlefield for recognition. The *Alien* movies (released in 1979, 1986, and 1992) presented an eerie metaphor for an unstoppable horror that surreptitiously enters, then grows inside the body, making a striking rhyme with the initial constructions of HIV. In each of these movies, a terrifying, virulently acid-based creature uses human beings as living incubators for her larvae. At the point of hatching, the maturing monsters literally rip apart their still-living hosts to be born. The living badness that was deposited in a human body for incubation is irrevocably and utterly destructive. The sequels elaborate fantasies of the ruthless mother determined to reproduce. In the sequels, the fantasy of the ruthless mother determined to reproduce is elaborated. The themes of maternal ambivalence, anxiety over narcissistic impingement in response to the process of childbearing, and fears of the terrifying bad mother are not to be neglected. What is compelling in the development of these themes as the cycle of films progresses is the dawning recognition of self in the heroine and the monstrous alien. Eventually, the heroine, Ripley, carries an alien embryo in her own uterus and destroys the newly delivered creature by killing herself as well as the alien. Recognition of the self in the other occurs at the moment of death. (Interestingly, the fourth film in the cycle, released in 1997, manifests the omnipotent syntax of the unconscious as Ripley is brought back to life: there is no death in the unconscious.)

A further resonance in this fantasy of becoming pregnant with a badness that will destroy its host is found in many gay men's responses to seropositivity. In significant ways, the emergence of the virus represented a massive change in the way gay culture had been constituted. As the decade after the Stonewall Riot unfolded, a gay male culture constructed itself around the celebration of newly claimed open attitudes about alternative sexuality. It is now almost a cliché to assert that during those years promiscuity became a political statement, as well as tantamount to the construction of identity. Any frenzied celebration expresses, among other things, a desperate attempt to exorcise, perhaps simply to ignore, what is dreaded and unwanted in the self. New Year's Eve, Mardi Gras, and Carnival are among the more organized of such functions. The celebratory hedonism of some parts of post-Stonewall gay life may have functioned in a similar way to expel the ubiquitous, loathed bad self that is the doppelganger of a gay consciousness. In addition, the necessary and painful mourning that Crespi (1995) has cited as required for the establishment of an identity other than one that is culturally sanctioned, may have been foreclosed or put off in those exhilarating days of sexual freedom. Established, organized prejudice has a paradoxically valuable function for a marginalized group: there is an armature on which to project the badness that cannot be acknowledged. This is in no way a suggestion that oppression is merely a projection; it is meant only to point out that among the many overdetermined responses to oppression, we can externalize and confront in our enemies what is loathsome to recognize in ourselves.

During the decade of the flowering of the gay movement as a political force, it became possible to build lives in openly gay environments. The gay ghetto became an identifiable area of many larger cities. Some gay men and lesbians were able to limit their social and professional contacts to other gay and lesbian people. Under such circumstances, the projected bad other could be more remotely externalized. Admission of shame and guilt concerning sexuality, and mourning the losses that establishing an alternative identity may involve, were elided in the ecstatic rush of sexual freedom. Like a developing virus, shame and guilt were hidden away until externalization stopped being an unconscious process and a metaphor. Illness became the mode of externalization: AIDS provided a newly constituted metaphor with physically palpable signs.

The power of the metaphor exploited in the *Alien* films is apparent in the return of the expelled bad other that is expressed in some gay men's constructions of their HIV infection. Shame and guilt, never far during even the most celebratory days of pre-AIDS gay culture, demanded recognition as HIV infection made its hosts pregnant not only with ripening infection, but with what had been expelled. In response to the desperate need of those suffering from an unthinkable terror, an industry arose among alternative healers to assist in the reintegration of this disavowed badness. Louise Hay (1986), a New Age healer, has been widely criticized for blaming the victims to whom she sold her balm. On the cassette recording of one of her soothing, meditative sermons, we were told that because gay men value beauty too much, we have been visited by a plague that leaves us disfigured and ugly. The way to redemption is to value our inner beauty. Her message not only established the guilt of the AIDS-affected community for their sufferings, but also implied that healing could occur once the guilt is embraced and the former hedonism is renounced. The polarities of the split are thus realigned, not in the interest of recognizing the self in the other, but as a means of casting out, once again, what cannot be tolerated. When the party ended, the celebrants became zealous penitents, and some eagerly embraced shame and guilt in an attempt to bargain away what had been psychic Otherness and was now a physical manifestation. A marketplace soon grew in which many varieties of reintrojection and reconstruction became available.

In the political arena, AIDS forced the gay community to coalesce into an effectively organized force, in a way that it had never before been able to organize itself. This has been regarded by many as a maturation of the gay community. Subsequently, dismaying reports of the rising incidence of risky sexual behavior have led others to lament that this represents an inability of many in the community to take responsibility for their actions. What must not be overlooked in this regard is the difficulty in experiencing oneself as an effective agent in one's life, in the circumstances the gay community has endured for the last two decades. Again, the issue of mourning emerges, as loss has explicitly become a universal experience.

Many seronegative gay men express incredulity as to why they have remained so. Often, they express the wish not to "be the last one left." Some are already the last of their chosen, self-constituted families. For many of these men, the difference between being negative and positive has meant that *their* needs, wishes, and fears have been neglected in the interest of caring for the sick and dying. To be seronegative thus becomes, in a paradoxical way, a burden; the seronegative becomes an Other, constituted by a negation. Antibodies to the virus have not been detected, and so these men have assumed a new name, the negatives (Odets, 1995). How does one stake a claim for one's own needs when designated a seronegative?[1] One answer seemed to be to subsume one's needs in the interest of those of the sick. Many seronegative men have spent nearly two decades working in the area of AIDS. Some skeptical and angry seropositives began to refer to such people as "AIDS vampires" in recognition of the apparent construction of an identity through the seropositivity of those for whom they cared. The struggle for recognition of the other is expressed in this symbiotic conflict, as each group constitutes the other, locating there its hatred and dread. We meet ourselves when we try to bridge the split between the positives and the negatives.

In the seropositive, the seronegative confronts himself. The transgressive means of exposure to the virus; the silent, invisible ripening of the disease; and the ultimate monstrous disfiguring course of the illness is a process that inherently declares the seropositive to be pregnant with the developing other—that is, disavowed—self, containing the shame and badness that the seronegative yearns and dreads to recognize.

---

[1] In the second decade of HIV/AIDS there were reports of "factitious" HIV infections. A small group of female patients was reported to have insisted that they were HIV positive, despite repeated tests indicating that they were not. As many of these women were often victims of physical and sexual abuse, we might speculate that claiming to be HIV positive was the only way for these women to obtain the help they knew they needed (see Mileno et al., 2001).

What happens when this monstrous pregnancy starts to show? At such a point, what has been known all along (perhaps) by one person is finally either revealed, or it is announced by obvious signs of physical deterioration. An identification will be made when it is articulated by the body that carries the virus. Is there value, then, in the notion or fantasy of establishing some kind of mastery over the mysterious entity that is invading one's cells while it still remains only an unknowable potentiality? For that is one of the defining factors of early-stage HIV seropositivity. After an initial bout of a flu-like condition, the newly converted seropositive generally does not notice anything amiss. The virus is most often knowable only by indirect, or surrogate, markers. It is not only not felt, but also difficult to observe directly in the host's bodily experience. (One of the significant clinical breakthroughs has been the development of the Polymerase Chain Reaction test that can measure the number of copies of virus per unit of blood. This is a more direct look at viral activity, yet it is still tantalizingly different from the direct observance of other manifest illness.) To claim this virus as an aspect of one's identity, or to have such an identity thrust upon one when serostatus is reported, alters fundamentally the relationships between the self and the body, and the self and mortality.

A common retort to the newly seroconverted person's concerns about a shortened lifespan is that none of us can ever count on not being hit by a bus while crossing the street. Of course, this retort is intended to be of comfort, but its effect is to widen the chasm between the one who is infected and the one who is not, instead of narrowing it. For, while it is true that none of us can really count on making it to bedtime alive, it is also true that most people do maintain a working conviction of life stretching on ahead of them. It is very easy to talk about the ease with which any of our lives could be ended when the conviction of life spinning out endlessly is not explicitly challenged. Those who suffer significant losses early in life are disabused of this fantasy, as is the person who receives a diagnosis of terminal illness. Psychoanalysts often meet them in consulting rooms, where the task is to convince them that they must dare to behave as if they believe their lives stretch endlessly before them.

The newly seroconverted HIV-positive man finds himself in a new, anomalous category. Though he may feel marked for death, superficially he is unmarked, except as he may designate himself. He is free of any sensations that intimate mortality yet is told that there is now cause for alarm and that the fantasy of uninterrupted life must be altered. Many have written and spoken of the remarkable gift this transition has turned out to be, how such a diagnosis provides the impetus to make life changes or to pursue goals with less conflict. Working through to a remarkable realignment of denial and acceptance, life is possible with a new, renegotiated balance between fantasy and dread. A healthy, crucial denial enables this process. At the same time, vital medical information—such as test results or studies of new drugs and their efficacy—must be assimilated, unimpeded by a need not to know and enabling the seropositive person to make important decisions. The loss of seronegativity comes with a terrible, urgent reminder of how much we take for granted. I have come to understand, more vividly than ever, that I contain that which will destroy me. I feel impelled now to name myself, rather than to allow myself to be named by others, passively, by default.

What, then, of the need of a seropositive person for a seronegative person? Is there a symmetrical bidirectionality in the yearning for recognition between us? The seropositive man has been seronegative, has known the fantasy of uninterrupted health, has been able to remain free of the dire choice of designating himself a site for recognition of the other. The seropositive may envy the seronegative's naiveté; in a crucial way, the seronegative embodies what is lost to him. I recall a flippant response among many gay men to the chilling calls for quarantine of all seropositives: that homosexuals were in quarantine already, at places like Fire Island and the other gay ghettos that developed following Stonewall. Those spaces claimed in a spirit of freedom could also work to isolate, a function prisons serve. This casual bravado expresses the knowledge that seronegatives use the presence of seropositives in the crucial project of maintaining a marked identity while struggling to recognize and not to recognize their *other*. Those who have been cast out already embody the split. Those who remain unmarked by otherness lack that knowledge.

THE HIERARCHY OF HIV INFECTION

It is tempting, but reductive, to discuss HIV infection only in terms of the binary of positive and negative. It was not until I found that I thought of myself as living in a different category that I understood how important that first category had been, and how important it is to further break down the binary at each step along the continuum of life with HIV. The categories have changed throughout my life: homosexual, HIV-positive, asymptomatic, long-term nonprogressor, needing medication, stable on the cocktail. With each category comes a new way of constructing myself, a new way of thinking about the various relationships that make up this life.

The most recent revision came about when my doctor proposed a vacation from medication. I had been on a triple drug cocktail: AZT, ddC, and Virimune, one of the nonnucleoside reverse transcriptase inhibitors. This regime initially was quite effective, driving my viral load below detectable levels of activity within six weeks. My T cells were in a normal range, well over twice the amount present when I first tested positive for HIV in 1989. In a few months, the viral load again became detectable, but at such a low level that it seemed safe to wait before changing the combination of medications. After six months and a steady upward creep in viral load readings, it seemed logical to establish a baseline of viral activity and to learn how effective the medication was. Four weeks after stopping all medication, my viral load was at a half million copies of viral RNA per cubic milliliter of blood. This was well within recent Centers for Disease Control (CDC) guidelines recommending treatment with protease inhibitors. My doctor suggested getting a confirmatory viral load reading, and two weeks later it was over 600,000 copies per unit of blood. It was time to join a new club.

How had I invented these factions of HIV positivity? The distress I felt indicated to me just how much I had invested in the condition of not needing the vaunted new medications, the ones that at first had tempted people to talk about "the end of AIDS." The longer I could avoid taking the latest drugs, the more data would be available to enable me to make informed decisions about them. But, in addition, there was a hierarchical structure among the seropositives that I had invented. Those at the top of the hierarchy are those who are seropositive but whose bloodwork shows no progression toward the development of AIDS. These people have a normal amount and ratio of T cells, and a reading of viral load shows no detectable replication of the virus. How do these lucky ones do it? It seems likely that they inherited a gene that prevents the human immunodeficiency virus from entering their cells and beginning its rapacious replication. Perhaps they were exposed only once to a relatively benign strain of the virus. It may be that their immune systems are exceptionally hardy and can produce enough T4 cells to mop up the 10 billion copies of the virus that flood their blood every day. Their apparently guaranteed survival of exposure to AIDS grants them their status at the apex of the positive hierarchy. A negotiation of an economy of stigma is detectable as well in that a moral valuation structures the hierarchy, too: the hardier, luckier ones may also be the better, more deserving ones.

Next comes those whose bloodwork remains very stable over long periods of time, who need only minimal medical intervention. This is the group in which I fancied myself. Perhaps it is more accurate to say that this is the group I invented for myself and then had to invent the others in order to situate my group in a context. There was a period of several years during which my membership in this group seemed unquestioned. This was a time when I could point to stress reduction, Chinese herbs, acupuncture, regular and reasonable aerobic exercise, and a prudent diet as sufficient to keep my HIV infection from progressing. The degree of mastery over the virus that I imagined was significant. At the second rung of the hierarchy, I learned that I had to master feelings of envy and guilt at not being as deserving of luck as those above me. So long as I did not require medication, I could maintain the necessary fiction that I was free of a life-threatening disease, and also that there were moral reasons why I was granted this relative good fortune, as well as reasons why I was shut out from the group above me. But if I was exemplary in my regime of self-care, I deserved my stable health. In time, that fiction was exposed as a lie, allowing the moral dynamic permeating this imaginary hierarchy to become apparent.

I did need medication, but (holding onto fantasy by my fingernails) I took solace in the fact that I only required the medications that had been around for a while: AZT and ddC. And then, I invented a new group in which to situate myself: those who do not suffer side effects of those drugs. If I could take them and not suffer, then I was in a location that felt a bit more privileged than that group who suffered headaches, gastrointestinal distress, neuropathy—all the accompanying reminders that one is taking what in the early years of its existence was an experimental drug that cannot cure, but does make one miserable. I was in this group for many years, and each slight adjustment of the medication regime seemed not to require the invention of a new group. Perhaps this was because there were new classes of drugs, each with its attending promises and failures, that formed new levels (into which I had not yet entered) of my hierarchy in the world of HIV.

It has been a relief that this world of otherness, populated with those marked by HIV, has become so fractured that in two decades of life with HIV/AIDS, it has lost its special status. Ironically, being marked by HIV emphasizes that any sense of being unmarked is ephemeral. Once a member of a group of *others*, the HIV-positive person is as much like, and as unlike, another HIV-positive person as anyone free of the virus is like, and unlike, him or her. The hierarchy of HIV infection, the splintering of an identity as HIV positive, simultaneously dissolves and maintains the boundaries of otherness.

A PSYCHOANALYST'S IDENTITITES

The psychoanalyst is the specialist of otherness. This is the role he or she assumes when taking up a position opposite the patient, or behind the couch. Poised between what is embraced and ejected, the specialist in otherness occupies a curious place, working to enable the recognition of the other. The question of the articulation of identity for the psychoanalyst who is HIV-positive is complicated because this dual status enacts the crisis that occurs as the cultivated invisibility, or opacity, of the traditionally constructed analyst is disrupted when his very physicality becomes a site for the struggle for the recognition of other. In that struggle, the boundary of the body becomes emphatically present, the intimation of a diseased physicality becoming a substantial impediment to the ideal of analytic transparency. Ironically and inevitably, when an illness of the body speaks for the therapist, the opaque veil of traditional analytic ideals is harder to hold in place.

Leo Stone (1961) asserts that "we cover our genitals and the greater part of our bodies except under special conditions; we do *not* usually cover our faces. . . . Actually, of course, the patient *does* see the analyst's face at the beginning and end of each hour; it is the psychological 'face' that we are prone to hide with what may often be over-wrought persistence and zeal [p. 50 emphasis in original]

Many disaffected potential analysands might regard "over-wrought persistence and zeal" as an understatement. There are many ways to hide one's face.

Maintaining an opaque identity in the interest of keeping the transferential field free of interference is a stance that has been critiqued among many groups of analysts (e.g., Aron, Benjamin, Hoffman, S. Mitchell, Renik). Isay (1996) describes the effects of his coming out as a gay man on the analyses of several patients. Showing his face by stating an aspect of identity led to new elaborations of transference, uncovering of new material, and often greater access to conflicted and repressed wishes. By steadfastly clinging to the belief that some activities are simple operating procedure whereas others amount to disclosures, analysts have seemed to wish that they may yet be able to control how they are to be constructed. We are now beginning to examine the meanings of such a wish.

Whether or not an analyst self-consciously articulates an identity, one is articulated for him or her. Of course, this is what analytic treatment is built on, the patient's articulation of an identity for the analyst constitutes the transference. In order to analyze, we must allow ourselves to be articulated.

Just as the heterosexual assumption was articulated when gay analysts began to come out, there is the HIV-negative assumption that prevents a patient from even asking an analyst about serostatus. Among that which is signified by the presence of HIV is sexuality (promiscuous, outlawed) and IV-drug abuse. (I neglect the "innocent" means of transmission, because such causes as blood transfusion might be considered to be more easily disclosed.) Any analyst would, I trust, welcome into the discourse with a patient any fantasy material concerning the analyst's engaging in outlawed behavior, as this would signify an important elaboration of the transference. But this development would occur well into treatment and would likely be predicated on the patient's conscious conviction that such a fantasy is far from the analyst's reality. What is initially assumed about the analyst is more often aligned with the ideal: that the analyst is contentedly married, stable in a richly rewarded and rewarding life. Indeed, how much pressure is felt by analysts to live up to these assumptions? How much anxiety is experienced by analytic candidates who do not fit such demographic idealizations?

We are here confronted with the question of how the category *identity*, initially an empty one, is filled. Postmodern theory has shown us the ways that identity is built through actions conscious or beyond awareness, and through the projective processes of others. The terms gay, HIV positive, and analyst, do not imply identity but require the hearing subject's interpretations and inventions of history. The act of signification fills the empty category. It is a daily and expectable affront to the therapist's narcissism that a certain amount of the signification of his identity is left for the analysand to make. The ways that the analyst is acted upon have been a traditional area of exploration. The ways that he or she acts are traditionally subsumed in what we know as technique. But this hardly exhausts the potential for a therapist's activity. What of the further action of signifying that the analyst is performed by? Regardless of theoretical allegiance, any psychoanalyst consciously or unconsciously chooses aspects of his or her life or character to reveal to patients. The manner of dress, style of office decoration, whether or not a wedding band is worn: all are consciously chosen disclosures (Goldstein, 1997). It may be argued that all the analyst's activity is in some way a disclosure (Renik, 1995b). He or she prepares, consciously or not, a characterization of self as analyst for presentation to the analysand. This very offering is an action, a communication, that has been theorized in various ways. Schafer (1983) has described a second version of the self that functions in the office: as analysts, we are better people than we ordinarily are. Winnicott (1951) described how analysts offers themselves to patients to be used in a new experience of object relating. Analysts who are concerned with questions of authority and power dynamics in the treatment dyad pointedly inquire into their patients' response to this presentation, so as to analyze the effect of such perceived power differentials in the treatment (e.g., Aron, 1996).

The analyst's preparation may have at least two components: readying the self to be used by the analysand, and creating a version of the self through the self-conscious activity of presentation. The stage is then set for the unfolding of the story the analysand and analyst will coconstruct. The analysis of this joint construction usefully employs the inquiry into the patient's fantasies about the analyst's subjectivity (Renik, 1995a, b; Aron, 1996).

Some analysts object to the constructivist stance, fearing that an emphasis on their subjectivity as a contribution to the treatment process will distract from or needlessly complicate analysis of patients' transference (Gabbard, 1996). In these warnings there is a determination to maintain a firm grasp on what is initiated by the patient, and what is added by the analyst, in the treatment relationship.

When I mentioned to a colleague that I was writing about what it is like to be an HIV-positive analyst, and about what happens when I tell patients that I am HIV positive, he replied, "Why would you tell a patient anything?" Clearly he advocates a stance in which it always clear what is whose in the analytic dialogue. When I heard this response, I recalled the first patient who asked me to disclose my serostatus to him. He felt that he could not work with a therapist who was not HIV positive. After acknowledging and exploring the element of extortion in his demand, I revealed my serostatus, and we began to work together. Eighteen months later, as he was talking about how ashamed he felt that he was HIV positive, he remarked that it was amazing that he could tell this to someone who was HIV negative. He had forgotten what had been so important before beginning treatment with me, and that I had in fact disclosed my status to him. This is an example of the power of the unconscious: when it was important for this man to feel different from me in this particular way, he forgot that it had once been crucial that we were the same, and to have my confirmation of that. He constructed me as he needed me to be.

Thus an identity can be seen to be an empty category prior to the coconstruction of relationships, and even afterward remains fluid according to the patient's constructions of the analyst. For this patient and this analyst, "HIV positive" functioned, at times, as an identity. In similar ways, the designation "gay man" serves a useful function, as does the appellation "psychoanalyst". What happens when a disclosure is made? An emptiness is filled, or a potential is foreclosed, but does this action deny the further elaboration of identity? The category is filled not by the HIV-positive person, not by the gay man, not by the analyst, but by the person who has heard the disclosure, by an interpreting subject.

In this way the transference of the psychoanalytic situation repeats what Foucault (1980) has theorized: that no identity is chosen—all are thrust upon us. We come into being through the exercise of power upon us in the process of "*assujetissement*," a term Butler (1997, p. 11) suggests we translate as "subjectivation." Foucault (1980) argues that

> The individual is not to be conceived as a sort of elementary nucleus, a primitive atom, a multiple and inert material on which power comes to fasten or against which it happens to strike, and in so doing subdues or crushes individuals. . . . The individual is an effect of power, and at the same time, or precisely to the extent to which it is that effect, it is the element of its articulation. The individual which power has constituted is at the same time its vehicle (p. 98).

It is secondarily that the subject interprets to himself the meaning of the identity that has been chosen for him. Lacan (1977) and others assert that our subjectivities are determined by our sex (Mitchell, 1982): we come into being as subjects by and through the establishment of sexual difference. But interpreting subjects need not remain stranded in the arid world of binary pairs. The experience of relating involves existing within the tension between the intrapsychic and the interpersonal, and sameness and difference assume an infinite number of possible meanings. The meaning that some individuals make of being HIV positive has to do with castration, with loss, with victimhood. Others have been able to create different and remarkably generative meanings for themselves. But the identity of "Other" is an inescapable shadow that is cast over the HIV-positive person from the moment of diagnosis.

I asserted that psychoanalysts are specialists in otherness. Perhaps I should say that I believe we ought to be, which is to say that otherness must by encompassed by the identity of psychoanalyst. So is "HIV-positive psychoanalyst" indeed an anomalous identity? This is contingent on the fashion in which the empty categories of identity are filled. Disclosure cannot exhaust the manner in which the infinitely capacious categories of identity can be elaborated. Actively filling in aspects of the identity as an analyst is in no way incompatible with the further project of psychoanalysis. It is an example of a subject's capacity for making meaning. One of the potential meanings has to do with the goal of confronting the otherness of the self. In the case of the HIV-positive person, that Otherness is often constituted by various configurations of sex and death. One goal of the recognition of the Other is to acknowledge the self-as-becoming, a turning away from the reified self that caught us all in the mirror. The self-as-becoming has limits, is separate, dies. The embrace of this becoming is the privilege and the privileged value of psychoanalysis.

CHAPTER 3

DISCLOSURE AND CONTAGION

WHEN MY LOVER DIED OF AIDS, our families immediately took in hand all the many things that needed to be accomplished in those first, blurred days. Among these was the matter of his obituary. I hesitated not a moment over whether to be listed as a survivor, although I was aware that several of the people I was treating at the time were themselves HIV positive or had lost someone they loved to AIDS, and so, like many of us, ritually scanned the obituary pages each day in a counterphobic accounting of AIDS deaths. The thought occurred to me that some patient would spot the obituary, identify me as his analyst, and wonder about my serostatus. But I did not hesitate to begin this process of potential disclosure. My decision to reveal an important, intimate fact about my life was folded into my desire to commemorate the relationship I had with the man I had cared for through his illness, who had died. But it is clear that the meanings of this decision are manifold.

I have been HIV positive for so long that, until the appearance of the protease inhibitors changed the lives of so many, for several years I was among those who annually stretched the period of time beyond the posited theory of the expectable progression to full-blown AIDS. Throughout my analytic training the irony of engaging in the intimate, long-term relationship of analysis as an HIV-positive person occurred to me, and I would spin out worst-case scenarios that involved the forced revelation to patients of an obvious, wasting, debilitating illness. Because I prize the transformative potential of mutuality, my fantasied revelation included my hope for mutual growth through the recognition of the patient's contribution to an important, real relationship. But it is noteworthy that in my fantasies I had to become ill in order for the disclosure to occur. My decision to be named in my lover's obituary countered the dreadful trajectory of my fantasy. It also led to a direct confrontation of how my disclosure affected my work with patients.

In my situation, the traditional notion of the transference becoming contaminated by any disclosure of mine felt particularly salient. In this way, the traditional analyst is like the HIV-positive person who guards his status in secret for as long as he can. There is destructive potential inside him, but as long as he maintains his secret and his distance, protecting the other from what is inside him, there is no risk of contamination. As long as the exchange does not involve body fluids, it is safe. Of course, by safe we mean that the transference will be more nearly isolated, readable, interpretable. In recent years, more and more analysts have dared to share coming out stories in which they recount how disclosures occurred and what happened (e.g., Davies, 1994; Frank, 1997). In contrast to a virus entering the bloodstream, the contamination of the transference has been shown to be inevitable, generative, and ultimately quite safe.

Before the death of my lover, I interviewed a prospective patient who had recently seroconverted. This was several years after the means of transmission of the virus were known, and, being in his fifties, and certain that he had practiced safe sex, he was extremely angry and ashamed of having seroconverted. He told me that he would not enter treatment with an analyst who was not HIV positive and asked me to reveal my serostatus. One way of thinking about his demand was to recognize his resistance to entering treatment. Some time ago, this man had completed a classical analysis lasting many years. That treatment, I was later to learn, was unsuccessful, as he continued to suffer from the feeling that he constantly played roles in an effort to accommodate himself to others (and had, in many ways, accommodated himself to his analyst, apparently with the analyst's support). In retrospect it seems clear that he needed to know that this treatment would be different. What kind of assurance about a new treatment experience could I offer? To what extent could we analyze his request that I reveal something of myself? I surely was being tested.

I responded that I understood how important it was for him to know for certain that I'd really know what it felt like to be HIV positive. This is arguably an appropriate response in such a moment, and one that can be made by any analyst, but there was also an element of masquerade inherent in my answer. This response held out the possibility that I was not HIV positive. Were I to explore the motivations behind his question without confirming or denying the truth, I would hold onto my option to maintain a falsehood. Undoubtedly there are compelling arguments for choosing this option. After all, it is the patient's needs that are the focus of the treatment, not the analyst's. Further, there will come a time when the patient wants his analyst to be seronegative. Then he will want to be certain that his analyst does not have needs that may supersede his own, that his analyst is not overwhelmed with anxiety and depression by his own potentially deteriorating condition. But is it not an equally false position to infer that, because any person is not HIV positive, that person will not be in a position to require care and attention? For surely this is an aspect of the fantasy communication, for both the sender and the recipient: "I will not reveal my status; your assumption that I am negative is correct." (For that is the assumption, I believe, that all patients make.) "I will survive and be sturdy and healthy and available to you no matter what."

So I told this man that I could understand the importance to him of my serostatus because I am HIV positive. And I found my eyes welling up with tears. I wonder now if I felt like crying for both of us, for this extraordinary situation we were in together. I had cried a great deal at the time of my testing for HIV. I had cried with each loss of a friend. I had cried in session with patients over terrible events in their lives, or at the termination of a treatment. But I was nearly crying at this moment for another reason—not out of sadness or mourning a loss, but out of something I had gained through the disclosure to this prospective patient.

Mitchell (1993) has pointed out that "[u]nderstanding does not provide much solace for, among other things, real loss, grief over lost opportunities, irreconcilable conflicts, and, ultimately, death. The analyst's understanding, no matter how powerfully transformative and also comforting it may be in some respects, is incapable of warding off or providing restitution for these losses, conflicts, and limitations" (p. 213). Perhaps we wept together in mutual acknowledgment of our inconsolable state: the uselessness of anyone's stating to us that they have some understanding about being HIV positive. My patient saw something of his experience in me, as I saw mine in him, and I joined him in working toward a recognition of our shared state by disclosing to him my status. But we also shared a private moment of acknowledgment that however much I can empathize, my understanding will still fail to ward off the dreadful inevitability of debilitating illness. Yet we agreed to work together. We persisted in maintaining a state of hope for transformation of some kind, though neither of us, I now believe, could have articulated then what that hope was.

Is it possible to say that I gained a different sense of authenticity through my disclosure? To assert this would imply that with all the patients to whom I had not disclosed this fact I had not been authentic. I do not believe this to be the case. But surely there is a particular experience of self-articulation that occurred for us both in the moment of disclosure. In one way, it would have been easy to frame this in terms of recognizing each other, as our situations mirrored each other's, and the question of sameness and difference. My patient was certain that if he were not in treatment with someone just like him, it would not work. At the same time, however, this man sought an HIV-positive therapist in order to exploit the differences between us; he hoped that my response to HIV positivity would be different from his. All this was articulated and elaborated as his treatment unfolded. But in that first session a process of self-articulation allowed both of us to recognize ourselves in a way that carried an unusual impact.

He told me he understood that it was unusual for an analyst to reveal any such fact about himself, expressing his gratitude that I had done so. What I came to know as his characteristic defensiveness dropped away for a time, as his need to recognize himself in the other in a concrete way was taken seriously. As our work progressed, I found little pressure to alter my technical stance in any way: there were no further disclosures on my part. When he asked me directly about my life, we were able to analyze the meaning of his requests. Vivid transferences emerged over time, which we both could play with and interpret. After three years, a new job took this man to a different city, and so a more complete analysis of the meanings of our shared status was not achieved.

Certainly important questions persisted regarding the meanings of my disclosure. A measure of skepticism about what is deliberately spoken is basic to our work. By this I mean that we reserve the right not to claim that we really know what and why we say anything, that there can always be more meanings to understand. The analyst who works with an asymptomatic HIV-positive client and asserts that the patient's seropositivity is not the central area of concern in analysis cannot help but hear the patient's material in a qualitatively different way from the material of a patient who is not HIV positive. Like any information one learns about a patient, it cannot be unlearned, cannot be left out of consideration. It becomes part of the narrative that is coconstructed in the analytic process. Similarly, knowledge of an analyst's seropositivity must alter the way that a patient chooses what to say, and how what the analyst says is heard; and it must also alter the patient's responses.

The HIV-positive analyst also hears a patient's material from a particular point of view. It is a point of view that may be helpful in becoming more empathically close to the patient, or it may make it extremely difficult to feel near to the patient's experience. But it cannot be neglected, it cannot be unlearned, the virus cannot be eradicated.

TYPICAL SCENES OF DISCLOSURE

In my practice, the disclosure of my serostatus typically came about in two ways. One was the scene in which a prospective patient sought out a therapist who was HIV positive. Since the incident I described at the beginning of this chapter, this scene has been repeated, though no patient has revealed my HIV status in making a referral. The other occurred when two patients I had been treating did, in fact, see the obituary of my lover and over time were able to ask directly about my serostatus. In their treatments, my disclosure exerted a number of effects. Existing transferences were intensified, and new or resisted transferences emerged in response to the information. Rather than limiting the kind of fantasy material or circumscribing a particular valence of emotional communication directed toward me, all of these areas, although undeniably affected by the disclosure, revealed new and heightened material.

KENT

Kent is a 44-year-old man whom I had been seeing for a month before he read the obituary in which I was named as a survivor of a partner who died of AIDS. Kent is himself a longtime asymptomatic HIV-positive man who came to this treatment (his third) depressed over the deaths from AIDS of most of his friends and two of his physicians. He was isolated, extremely passive, and presented himself as unable to do anything for himself. He was filled with shame over his perceived inadequacies and had felt ashamed since his childhood. His severely depressed father had had a history of multiple psychiatric hospitalizations and had been arrested several times for soliciting sex in highway rest stop men's rooms. Kent's parents were Southern Baptists, and homosexuality was a grievous sin to them. Shame about the father's homosexuality poisoned the lives of the entire family. Kent had found no acceptable way to express anger other than in a passive–aggressive style, which could, at times, be quite provoking. It seemed to me that he used others to contain feelings of rage that he could not tolerate in himself. There was also a tremendous conflict between his wishes to depend on another and his fears of what would be repeated if he were to depend on another.

When I telephoned Kent to inform him that a death in my family had occurred and that I would not be seeing patients that week, he told me that he had read the obituary and offered his condolences. He asked if there was anything he could do for me. When I returned to work, he reiterated this offer. Kent found the role of caring for others much more congenial than asking directly for anything for himself. We learned that he felt that, if he could perform some caretaking task, then the cared-for person might reciprocate. All relationships entailed this sort of quid pro quo. Underlying his solicitousness was concern for my physical health. He repeatedly said that he felt that his need to talk about his own health concerns would be harmful to me and evoked the possibility of losing another person. He admitted that he fantasized that talking about his own seropositivity would make me get sick, and he could not stand to lose someone else. He asked me to tell him if it was all right with me for him to talk about HIV concerns and added that he would-n't take it personally if I told him I couldn't work with him any longer. His fears about my ability to withstand his aggression and dependence had roots both in his current situation and in his history. In the weeks that followed, Kent stated that he felt self-conscious complaining about anything, since I had just lost my lover. He struggled with the question of whether or not treatment could be helpful to him at all. His fears about my inability to withstand his complaints or neediness suggested to me that he had reached some conclusions as to my health based on the information he'd learned about me. In the first several months of our work I repeatedly pointed out the theme of his difficulty in trusting that I'd be reliable, able to tolerate all of his feelings and needs. But I felt that there was another question that Kent was trying not to formulate—the question of my seropositivity.

Nearly a year and a half later, the anniversary of his physician's death, Kent reported his most recent bloodwork results and added that he was concerned about my health. He thought that I had lost weight recently and observed that I was looking tired. The worry that his needs would be too much for another person to handle motivated his questioning. His knowledge of my lover's death provided a means for the direct expression of these fears. The anniversary of the death of his doctor was the impetus he needed to ask me directly about my serostatus. I responded by asking if this question had been on his mind for a long time. He said that it had but that it had not seemed to him to be possible for him to ask: "It didn't seem like it was any of my business." I pointed out that he had lost two doctors, as well as many friends, so such a question was most certainly his business. He replied that his seeing me as an authority figure prevented him from asking me direct questions most of the time. I wondered openly if his repeated concerns about my ability to tolerate his neediness also prevented him from asking about my serostatus. He agreed that it had. I asked what it would be like for him if I were HIV positive. He said that he would be sad but that it wouldn't make any difference now about his decision to work with me.

The moment had come for me to confirm his long-standing suspicion. Though he had told me that he'd feel sad if I were HIV positive, it was obvious that there were other, unformulated feelings about my seropositivity. I had speculated to myself that a part of Kent would be quite satisfied if he knew that I was, and that he needed to work very hard to keep this voice from being heard, either by himself or anyone else. But it was clear to me that his treatment would continue to unfold regardless of what I told him, and that the ways Kent organized our relationship would indeed be affected according to my answer. So the question came down to my sense of how I wished to make myself known to him.

The relationship between us had been contaminated since he had read the obituary in the paper. That contaminant had served to accentuate and emphasize aspects of Kent's style of relating, but it also echoed the ways in which Kent experienced himself as contaminated. I was now contemplating naming myself as contaminated in the same way. I believed that Kent knew the answer to his question already. Was the confirmation of my seropositivity best conceptualized as countertransference acting out? Viewed from this perspective, my telling him this fact could be interpreted in many ways: as a counterphobic attempt to demonstrate that no matter what, I would be hardy enough to tolerate his needs; in a hostile/competitive demonstration of how much better I was at managing my health than he was; as a way to undermine his idealization of me as an authority figure. But what is the risk of contamination? Were any of these possible themes made less analyzable or potentially useful in my work with Kent following my confirmation of his suspicion?

One way of approaching this question is to consider whether it is the content of a disclosure or the process leading to and from a disclosure that inhibits or promotes analytic work. For example, a major theme in our work had been his style of relating. Passive–aggressive was a label that Kent himself had affixed to his behavior, and he recognized it as a way to try to elicit a particular response from others, including me, without appearing to be demanding. He had described how others had identified his characteristic style of self-presentation as indicating that he was too weak to defend himself, so that he could make covert attacks without fear of retaliation. It could be reasonable to interpret my disclosure as a retaliation of my own, in a similarly passive–aggressive style. It is entirely likely that a similar kind of countertransferential retaliation could be made with different content. In either case, a different response to Kent's wondering, such as an interpretation of aggressive or destructive wishes, if the timing had been right, was forestalled. So I told him.

> GC: Well, I want to let you know that I am HIV positive.
> K: How are you doing? Your numbers. Are you on medication? Is—is it all right to ask?
> GC: Well, what I'd like to tell you is that I've been positive since before 1982, that I'm lucky enough to not need medicine at this point, and that I've never had an opportunistic infection . . . How is it for you, that I've let you know all this?
> K: Thank you for telling me. I'm glad you're doing well. I've wondered; I think I knew before now. But I didn't . . . I didn't think you'd tell me.
> GC: Why wouldn't I?
> K: Because . . . to keep a distance.
> GC: From you?
> K: From all your patients.
> GC: You especially?
> K: I'll have to think about that.[1]

---

[1] Material from sessions with patients is reconstructed from notes made after the sessions were over.

Through my confirmation, I spoke directly to Kent's positioning himself toward me as a subordinate who has no rights in our relationship, and this opened into an exploration of that theme. In retrospect, I believe that if I had remained opaque and chosen not to disclose my serostatus, this may have amounted to a confirmation of Kent's experience of himself as having no rights.

But what of the content of Kent's fantasies about me, with regard to the potential of interpretations I might make in the future? Now that I had revealed myself as contaminated, how was our relationship different? Many potentialities were positive: knowledge of our shared serostatus might effect a change in his idealization of me, which I experienced as working to maintain distance between us. Erotic fantasies, triggered by Kent's seeing me as a sexually active person, could become more prominent. Perhaps seeing me as flawed in some way could lead to a greater prominence and ease of expression of more overt aggression in Kent's material.

In this light, I thought of how Kent seemed unconsciously to claim responsibility for the deaths of his doctors and friends.

Shortly after I made my disclosure, Kent reported a disturbing memory of a recent Fourth of July Party. He and a group of friends had a picnic on the roof of a friend's building that had a great view of the fireworks on the river. One of the group was a man who was quite ill with AIDS. Kent told me that he had felt gripped by the impulse to push this man off the roof of the building. He could not imagine why he'd have such a feeling, and said that he felt extremely upset and guilty.

I wondered whether my disclosure of my status, which he regards as highly stigmatic, could have been linked to this most vivid and explicit emergence of aggressive material. Often before it had seemed as though Kent felt responsible for the deaths of other friends, and we had connected this to his worries that talking about his concerns would be harmful to my health. But this memory was the first example of explicitly aggressive material that Kent was able to tell me. Was there a way that his knowledge of my tainted condition enabled him to tell me about aspects of himself that he was frightened and ashamed of?

At this point in our work, Kent began dreaming intensely, bringing in many dreams that he spent the bulk of our sessions describing and interpreting. He expressed a good deal of satisfaction in exploring his dream material, and it was clear that, despite his stated apprehensions about my ability to be reliable, he had become able to use our relationship in a more intimate way. As Kent's involvement in his unconscious material grew, we both agreed that use of the couch and increased frequency of sessions would be helpful. One way that I sensed Kent's growing use of me as an object was my own greater ability to recognize and eventually interpret my presence in unconscious derivative material, such as his dreams, in ways that were expressive of crucial self and object representations.

One dream took place at a flea market that was in the same neighborhood as my office. He was there with a companion whom he could not identify. They went into one booth that sold various Asian food stuffs and other items. An old woman sat near a large tub over which hung a large shark, so that the shark's head dangled behind and above her. From time to time, the shark took bites out of her head. Among Kent's associations to this dream was the connection he made between the spatial relationship of the woman and the shark, and the way it resembled his relationship on the couch to me, seated above and behind him. This was the first time he was able to identify his fears and anger with me for "taking bites out of his head"—intruding with my endless quest to understand what he had to say to me. Perhaps this dream also expressed something of his response to my contaminated state, that I was dangerous and hostile.

It would be difficult to argue that Kent's becoming a good patient had to do with my disclosure of material that represented an aspect of the lived, extraanalytic experience that we shared. I believe that far more was accomplished with my disclosure than was sacrificed. But whether the content of the disclosure was as important as the process of disclosing is a subtle question. Surely Kent and I seek to recognize in each other some fears about HIV infection and fantasies of the living badness we each have inside us. This content-related experience is unique to the dyad where HIV infection is disclosed. We differ, and have made explicit how we differ, on our expectations about our futures. In this Kent looks to me, as did the patient I described earlier, for a model of how to hope for a future that is different from progressive debilitation and death at an early age.

In retrospect, it feels slightly ironic to refer to the hope that I, as analyst, held out to this patient. But this is undoubtedly what I do whenever I meet a new patient. There were many times when I felt pressured to actively assert an alternative point of view about HIV infection with Kent. It is curious to me that on this topic I felt far less constrained from activity than with other material. Mitchell (1993) pointed to the distinction between hope in a state of mind dominated by a longing for an omnipotent, magical, easily controllable object, and hope in a state of mind where the wished-for other is acknowledged to be an only human, irreplaceable, uncontrollable object. "To keep an analyst's offer of hope alive long enough to be useful and genuinely nourishing requires the precarious suspension of the complementary, comfortably foreclosing processes of idealization and envy" (p. 212).

My disclosure came at a time when Kent required that I be omnipotent, magical, and easily controlled. I believe that here lies one clue to where I felt I could be active and where I could wait. Our shared knowledge about each other admitted death to our relationship as an active partner. I felt that I had to fight for both of our lives at times, to fight in order to maintain the space for both of us to have life, potential, time. Of course my fight exploited Kent's hope for the omnipotent object that could magically take away the virus inside him. In order to fight for the potential of the treatment I had to exploit my own hope for just such an omnipotent object. Far from indicating a trap to be avoided, this provides a profoundly intimate foundation for a transformative experience. The way that we share a state of consciousness in which we depend on fantasies of rescue and deliverance does not mitigate against our finding ways of relating without reliance on fantasies of omnipotence, idealization, and envy. It creates the contrasting ground against which to find that other way of relating. It may be that a reasonable statement of the hope that an analyst holds out to a patient would include this possibility of finding an alternative point of view.

Most patients, I believe, see such an option as based on lived experience. I am reminded of jokes among several analyst friends about our envy of patients who have more fully realized lives than we do. Whose lived experience would be emulated by whom? So once again we confront the ways fact and fantasy in regard to the analyst's presentation converge and diverge, and, what was more painful for me to understand, the ways the hopes and fears of the analyst and the patient converge and diverge.

For years into the treatment, our positions with regard to hope and lived experience were tested. Kent's routine blood work indicated a decrease in his T cells and an increase in the viral load as measured by the Polymerase Chain Reaction (PCR) test. His doctor recommended that he begin taking one of the protease inhibitors that had only recently become available. This involved Kent's starting AZT again, a medication that he had taken for several years and that left him anemic and feeling generally terrible. (Protease inhibitors are administered in conjunction with two of the reverse transcriptase inhibitors such as AZT or 3TC, in a sort of cocktail to attack the virus at two points in its life cycle.) Kent immediately began talking about the discomfort he was experiencing from being on AZT again, and especially about the constraints that the protease inhibitor placed on him. For this protease inhibitor to be optimally effective, a strict dosage schedule had to be rigorously followed: it had to be taken one hour before eating, two hours after having eaten anything, and every eight hours. At first glance, this may seem a not unreasonable dosage schedule to maintain. But on reconsideration, it is clear that this limited the patient's options to a considerable degree. If the dosage schedule was, say, 7:00 A.M., 3:00 P.M., 11:00 P.M., lunch must be finished, every day, by 1:00 P.M., and dinner by 9:00 P.M. We were cautioned that missing or delaying a dose risked having the level of drug in the blood dip below a certain threshold, and that this would enable the virus to become resistant to the drug, apparently permanently. Once the virus adapts to the reduced level of drug in the blood, it can remain impervious to even higher levels of drug; further, cross-resistance to other protease inhibitors was shown in early studies of the drugs. All this was understandably anxiety provoking. The protease inhibitors were the first major clinical breakthrough in a long time. The studies that led to their approval by the Federal Drug Administration (FDA) indicated that this new class of drugs reduced viral load to below detectable levels in the study subjects and raised T cell levels significantly, for the duration of the studies in some subjects. This was the most encouraging news about the treatment of HIV in the history of the epidemic. Doctors now conjecture, with more confidence than ever before, that HIV infection could become a treatable chronic condition, and that seropositive individuals may be able to enjoy a more normal life span. (Since the time of the sessions summarized here, protease inhibitors and other HIV/AIDS medications have been formulated to make them far easier to take.)

I present this in such detail because I was lucky enough, at that time, to have waited a considerable period—during which the various protease inhibitors were tested and more data accumulated—before needing to start this new medication regime. As long as my blood work indicated that I was remaining stable, I could maintain the denial that had permitted me to work with so many sick people while HIV positive. Around the time Kent started his protease inhibitor, I had bloodwork done as well, and the question as to whether I would start a different medication regime arose once again.

As Kent expressed, in his characteristically mild and singsongy way, his dismay over the problems of taking his medication, I found myself becoming more and more agitated. Often I work until 9:00 P.M. and eat dinner after that. I began trying to figure out what kind of dosage schedule would work for me, should I have to begin taking this protease inhibitor. My family lives on the West Coast: what happens when one travels across time zones? How is travel to Europe possible while one maintains a strict dosage schedule?

As I listened to Kent, I felt myself rebelling against the roles we had coconstructed, which were determined significantly by my disclosure of seropositivity. How I longed for a way to deny all that was happening to both of us. How I hated feeling that Kent needed me to maintain my optimistic, reasonable state of mind, confident that he would find a way to make the dosage schedule work, ready to analyze the process unfolding between us. His underlying resistance to taking these medications was contagious. No! I wanted him to shut up, because his concerns were intruding on my precariously maintained optimism about my own potentially imminent need for this medication. I realized that, despite my disclosure, Kent and I both needed, from time to time, to forget that I was HIV positive.

Once the disclosure had been made, we both seemed to be drawn inexorably toward denial of the disclosed content. I think this points to questions of hope in the analytic situation. Kent idealized me, as analysands do, in order to believe that a point of view different from his about himself was possible. The problem of how to live with being HIV positive is a crystallization of this dynamic. On several occasions, Kent asserted that we who are seropositive could have no hope for a normal life span, or even a reasonably happy shorter one. In such moments, it is clear to me that I am the repository for any hope for a life that can include happiness, sexual satisfaction, intimacy. In order to maintain this status, I am seen as free not only of the fatalism that dominates Kent's bleak point of view, but also as free from the doom that being HIV positive has always meant. We each in this way deny that I am really HIV positive.

Were I not, would this scenario be altered altogether? Were I to be seronegative, there would be concrete proof of the dissonance between our points of view and experience. How easy it would be to see my blithe maintenance of hope that Kent can experience good things in life as based on an utter lack of understanding of his condition. When I refer to a blithe maintenance of hope, I refer not to anything I may have said or done in our work, but to the position in which our mutual construction of our relationship might have placed me. By reserving my option of having a different point of view about life as an HIV-positive person, whether or not I have confirmed my serostatus in a relationship with Kent, has meant that I have hope that life can include happiness while he does not. To maintain an abstemious, neutral (uncontaminated and uncontaminating?) posture does not guarantee being perceived as remaining neutral as to the outcome of analytic work. At the very least, analysts are hopeful that neurotic or characterological suffering can be transformed into ordinary human suffering.

Which leads to the impossible question of what can be called ordinary about the suffering in the condition of being ill. What is a nonneurotic response to one's seroconversion? Until quite recently, most people were told that they could look forward to 5 to 10 years of healthy life. This estimate is stretched annually as more and more people live longer. With the introduction of new medications, some are boldly predicting 20 years or more of AIDS-free life. All through the epidemic, the long-term nonprogressors have been a small group whose experience has not been widely known or disseminated. Has this been so as not to arouse unrealistic hopes? The point is that the nonneurotic response to seroconversion is an impossibly idealized acceptance of the unalterable condition of us all: that we have no reasonable justification for counting on anything about our existence. This confrontation leads to the process of renouncing omnipotence. Is this a confrontation that can be experienced imaginatively? Empathically? Or must it be lived through?

The sense of nonattachment that works as a fulcrum point in eastern meditative practices might be thought of as such a renunciation. The relative success of the Bodhisattva's progress toward nonattachment is based on the belief that the life we are limited to knowing is an illusion, a meaningless cloud to be passed through on the way to ultimate enlightenment and attainment of Buddha nature. Acceptance of human fallibility and limitations through analysis, on the other hand, is not based on convictions of spiritual or religious belief. Accepting our own limitations and humanity depends on our having accepted the limitations and humanity of our caregivers. This necessary, inevitable disillusionment is what eventually allows us access to a nuanced understanding of the subjectivity of the other and the acceptance of difference (Benjamin, 1995). And this requires knowing that we are already contaminated, contaminated with humanity. Disclosed information is potential evidence of the independent subjectivity of that other, as is the open assertion of a differing point of view.

Maintaining a different point of view from that of Kent involves walking the narrow path of believing that we legitimately can determine something about the quality of our lives, while seeking to remain more nearly free of the sway of omnipotent fantasy in doing so. What is the process whereby we differentiate hope from omnipotent fantasy? For anyone who is HIV positive, hope boils down to what certainly *is* omnipotent fantasy: a cure; a way to undo what has been done; a way to remove something that has become part of our bodies and is growing within lymph glands, macrophages, T cells, testicles, breast milk, and vaginal secretions, even inhabiting our brains. To have hope is to rely on that which is assuredly impossible. Yet how do any of us who are HIV positive function without such omnipotent fantasies?

As Kent's treatment continues, among the potential selves and others that Kent and I present for each other are two parallel tracks along which the relationship between us has unfolded. One is the extraordinary track of our shared knowledge and experience of each other as HIV-positive people. The other is the ordinary track of a treatment in which Kent presents himself to his analyst for help. Throughout a given session, the parallel tracks merge, and, as I have described, there is an ironic switch in our roles as to who holds the hope in our relationship. Another way of describing this process may be that those moments are the ones where I can identify my denial breaking down, where I no longer can rely on omnipotent fantasy to support me in our quest to outgrow omnipotent fantasy. The paradox is inescapable. My ability to sustain an omnipotent fantasy functions in the service of analytic work with Kent, whose aim is a way of functioning free of omnipotent fantasy and the attendant dread of its failure. When I fail to sustain an omnipotent fantasy, when my denial of what is true about me breaks down, it is the mutually constructed creation of me as Kent's analyst that sustains us. Mutual construction is a form of contagion. I use this term on purpose to emphasize that I recognize problematic as well as beneficial aspects in every choice I've made in my work. At a point like this, when I feel unequal to the task of maintaining a reliable sense of my robust vitality, I must rely on Kent's idealization, envy, and denial that have created the role of analyst to restore my function as the keeper of the hope that another point of view is viable.

Is one moment any more authentic than another, along what I've reified into two parallel tracks? Or is the question rather whether one mode of functioning, as reflected in the particular moment, is more helpful to the patient than another? As the question of the needs of the patient are ascendant, we run headlong into the false dichotomy between the patient's needs and the authenticity of the analyst's presentation of himself. Ferenczi (1932) already did the research for us on the potential of the analyst's expression of his vulnerability, fear, and fantasy. He abandoned his experiments in mutual analysis because he and his patients were driving each other crazy. But in a more nearly conventional analytic situation, the easy answer is that it doesn't matter what is more helpful to a patient because moments such as the one I am trying to describe are inevitable in any treatment, regardless of the real-life conditions of the participants.

I did not express any of the feelings I experienced as Kent described his apprehensions and anger over his new medication regime. It remained for me to explore the potential meanings of the feelings I experienced before bringing them into the work in some way, if at all. Clearly this material is analyzable, useful counter-transference. Invoking this term, I must include this association: it is as if a shroud is cast over my recollection of the relationship with Kent, as if there is a closing-off of exploration by using this word. In a sense, I am battling my analytic-culture superego, constituted by and constituting a fantasy of the impossibly idealized analyst who never discloses, is always ultimately helpful to patients, and who remains pristine. This imago is also surely free of HIV.

We lived through our phase of mutual contagion; the matter of my seropositivity receded into the background of the treatment; and Kent's did too. Eventually, death appeared as a dynamic theme from a time in Kent's life predating HIV infection and in intimate association with depression and the family history. One day in the sixth year of our work, Kent began to describe the fragments of what felt to him like a memory of a fantasy, or a waking nightmare, that had troubled him since he was a young boy of about five or six. He told me that he thought it was based on a horror movie he'd seen, but he couldn't recall. As he spoke, there was the unmistak-able sense that, with each word, more of the fantasy became clear. This was new material in our work.

In his fantasy, he was a prisoner who devised a scheme to escape from prison, with the help of an accomplice. He and the accom-plice would pretend to die and would be buried. Then, after the guards had left the gravesite, the two men were supposed to dig themselves out.

> "I'm buried alive. In order to escape, the other guy, my accomplice, is supposed to wake up and help me dig us out. I look over and it's my father—and he's not just sleeping, he's dead. I remember that his hand is like a skeleton. It's horrible. I'm a little boy, buried alive, next to my dead father." [He was sobbing, breathless.]

Articulating what appeared to be an unconscious fantasy that had organized much of Kent's experience precipitated a lifting of his depression. He described a space opening up between his own torso and a "shadow" that used to fill and cover him at the same time. Shadow was his term for his depression; it was more a somatic sensation, a cold numbness, than a visual metaphor. For some time it had seemed as if the shadow was HIV, but now he realized that the shadow had been there long before his illness. He eventually came to identify the shadow as his father. The childhood fantasy of being buried alive with his dead father, a father who was dead with depression when he was alive, dead to his family because of his homosexuality, had been transformed into a somatic trace memory, a fantasy of death in life worn in and on his body.

HIV had absorbed, taken on, and imparted a name to an experience that had somatic presence but was mostly lived as depression. When the fantasy could be put into words, this system was reorganized. HIV lost its power to explain everything, and Kent's sense of himself as interpreter of his experience grew. What became clear was how he had created a way of understanding his shame, anger, and sadness. As a defense against knowing them, he had translated these feelings into an inscrutable language of mood and vague bodily experience. This fantasy was available for HIV to take over, to infect, almost in the same manner in which the virus can enter and take over cells of our immune systems. This fantasy was also useful in describing a quality of our relationship, those despairing, helpless moments when Kent could not imagine my truly being alive. In recovering this fantasy, Kent was able to suppress the virus in the interest of our analytic work, making room for his life again.

The relief brought by articulation of this fantasy opened the way to a rediscovery of Kent's love and talent for painting and drawing, which led to his daring to express himself more vigorously. Kent told me that he'd won an award in junior high school for his drawing, but that it had never seemed to be a talent he ought to take seriously. It was around this time that Kent began to take classes in drawing, painting, and printmaking. Soon he had rearranged the furniture in his apartment to create a studio. His enthusiasm and his confidence in the rediscovered talent grew. He told me: "On the way down to this session today, I was . . . I was crying . . . growing tearful, for some reason. I was feeling so happy that I started to cry. It's all right, I'll turn into a leaky faucet for good things, too . . . I feel so much energy inside me, but it's energy I can *use*, it doesn't use me. Before, it was as if it was bound up in depression. Now I can . . . I was going to say . . . play with it. Now I'm feeling—emotional."

So was I. For Kent to say that he could now *play* was one of those triumphs that are precious and rare in our work.

*   *   *   *

When I gave Kent an early version of this chapter to read, he pointed out that I had not included a consideration of my experience of the deaths of patients who had AIDS. It was rather shocking to have this brought to my attention because several patients have worked with me through the last stages of their illnesses. Our work involved hospital visits, collateral meetings with their caregivers, sessions at their homes when they were too ill to leave their beds. As I wondered about this omission, I realized that these were the moments when it was absolutely required of me that I bracket my own seropositivity, in order to be as present as I could possibly be for these men. Kent's worry, that if he were to get sick I'd be overwhelmed, is answered in this recollection. I wasn't overwhelmed when I thought about my work because my defenses were effective enough to allow me to continue working as an analyst. It was possible for me to see myself at these last stages of AIDS only after each patient's death, in my private grieving and fear.

As to Kent's having mentioned this, I was cheered by his ability to point out an omission as glaring as this. In a way, his use of our work together is illustrated by this moment in which he made himself more of a collaborator in this project.

JASPER

The other patient who read my late lover's obituary and wondered about my health is an HIV-negative man whom I'd been seeing for two years. Jasper had been in treatment before, for five years, and had found it of limited use, though his obsessive thoughts and compulsive behaviors had, to a significant degree, diminished. By the time he began to work with me, he had been in a gratifying committed relationship with his partner for eight years and had established himself in a successful career in a highly competitive and stressful field. Typically, he required little from me in terms of verbal contribution in our time together. I found it very easy to listen to him, as he is a charming raconteur with a lively sense of humor. I understood that Jasper needed me to admire and celebrate his growing capacity to tolerate frustration and solve difficult problems with skill and élan, an experience of having his strivings and successes acknowledged that he had missed throughout his life.

I received a card of sympathy from Jasper in the week following the appearance of the obituary. The next time we met for a session, three weeks later, he told me about the friends he had lost, and one in particular whom he helped to look after through several hospitalizations. He said that he'd never want to live through that again. I heard quite clearly his wish that I not give him any bad news about myself. In the several months that followed, Jasper seemed more pointedly to fill our hours with events from his daily life. I inquired as to whether he was avoiding asking me about what he'd learned concerning me from the obituary of my lover. Over and over again he told me that he did wonder about me but was not ready to ask directly, and that I shouldn't make him ask.

We remained in this odd embrace of knowing but not knowing for several months. Throughout this time, Jasper's material included concerns about my ability to keep up with him, to withstand his angry or sad feelings, his criticisms of me. Finally I pointed out to him that he was, in effect, asking me the question he had determined that he could not formulate: that about my serostatus. He agreed that he was wondering but had hoped that he could conclude treatment without asking about it. He added that my bringing it up brought to mind an early memory: on a family visit to his grandmother of whom he was afraid, he refused to get out of the car. His father had to drag him from the car, crying and struggling to stay inside. He easily interpreted this memory as referring to his wish that I not make him know what he already knew but wished not to.

Jasper stayed in that car most of the time. This was his method of protecting himself against what he experienced as overwhelming compulsions that had, in the past, ruined his life. From my point of view, the problem was the way this metaphor had metastasized. In treatment, Jasper had made it clear that he sought not to discuss his former compulsions, because he was managing them with relative success and felt resigned that his more or less effortful management of himself would be a condition of his life forever. As our work continued, it became apparent that his management style of keeping himself in that car inhibited other areas of relating, particularly when it came to feelings of closeness that were not sexual, as well as sexual fantasies and angry feelings, which frightened him. The possibility of exploring sexual feelings in the transference was out of the question. Jasper explained that he was confident that I would maintain an appropriate boundary if he were to describe his affectionate and erotic feelings for me, but that he was terribly anxious about what it would feel like for him afterward, when he left my office. It was as if talking about sexual wishes would weaken his resolve to maintain his sexual sobriety outside.

I wondered if he felt that having one erotic thought bred an unquenchable fever of impulse that would infect me as well. Was he afraid that neither of us could be safe from that erotic infection, so the only way to stay safe was to avoid contact with any of what must be, for analysts, the juicy parts, the "body fluids" that carry such affective and infectious power? So I asked him if he felt that his sexual thoughts could be contagious and that we would be unable to keep ourselves from acting on them. He admitted that he did fear such a possibility. It became apparent that a significant portion of Jasper's inner world was off limits to us. It was a striking irony that it was Jasper who experienced himself as containing the infectious contagion. Yet the question remained as to whether and how my disclosure may have contributed to this phobic avoidance. Did I now present to him the image of someone who must pay for his impulses with HIV infection?

Nearly two years after the death of my lover, Jasper decided to terminate our work together. He suggested a three-month period of time to work through our ending. At first, I agreed that terminating was an appropriate move. In all areas of his life, Jasper was able to derive great satisfaction, this in spite of having to cope with the hospitalization of his mother and other difficult events. Through all this, Jasper told me about his satisfaction in his relationship and his confidence that his career was moving in a progressive direction, and he described many important friendships. He was experiencing a rich life. Therapy had been helpful. Jasper said that he was grateful, but he thought it was time to move on. How could I not agree?

And yet . . . and yet. . . . I was not certain that I could endorse our termination, when this would mean ignoring that significant portion of Jasper's inner life that was forbidden to me. I felt left out, cheated, and guilty: cheated because we had not been able to address the erotic transference, guilty that Jasper's response to my serostatus was part of what created the terra incognita that we were both to ignore.

So I objected. I told Jasper that I had changed my mind about ending and explained why. I told him I was uncertain exactly how and why the revelation of my serostatus had inhibited our ability to address some important feelings and fantasies, but I knew that it had. I explained that I could not be comfortable with an ending that left so much unsaid. Jasper emitted what I heard as a deeply felt sigh of recognition and agreed. But, he protested, it was impossible for him to imagine talking about compulsive behaviors with someone whom he did not know for sure had struggled with compulsive behaviors in his own life. He was certain that I could not ever really understand. For Jasper, the frightening aspect of our situation was the living badness inside of *him*. We seemed to be locked in an ironic embrace of mutual not knowing. I held open the possibility that my disclosure took on certain meanings for him and explicitly wondered if HIV represented, to him, the consequences of compulsive sexuality. Jasper denied this, insisting that he felt no judgment of me, only regret. His denial strengthened my belief in my conjecture. But that is where we were stuck. If my disclosure had taken on meanings for Jasper about my impulsivity, we would have to find the words to speak it, to get out of the car. But that felt like risking being swept away in the torrent of impulse that waits outside of it.

At that point, I was pulled up short. When other patients had protested that I could not possibly understand something unless I had actually experienced it, it was about their experience of being HIV positive. This struggle over sameness and difference is part of every treatment. Those who experience themselves as opposed to or barred from alignment with the symbolic order of patriarchy often find it difficult to begin treatment with someone they assume *is* in a position of alignment. HIV is another marker for the Other who is removed from or defiant of the symbolic order. The seropositive patient who seeks an HIV-positive analyst, the gay patient who seeks a gay therapist, the compulsive patient who needs to know if his therapist has struggled with compulsions, all experience themselves as unable to negotiate the schism between positions that are either sanctioned or not by the symbolic order.

As I have described, the question of difference emerges in spite of my disclosure, as it will no matter what is disclosed. Metaphors for difference will insist on making their presence known because the acceptance and reconciliation with difference is one of the most important opportunities that treatment offers. The ironic and perplexing face-off between Jasper and me had to do with this problem of sameness and difference. I wish to point to a potential mutuality of our perceptions of ourselves: that we each have an experience of containing that which will destroy us.

But Jasper could not permit himself to move that close to me. It may be that by staying inside the car, he avoided encountering his dreadful fears that he was as incomprehensible to another as he was to himself. Perhaps his feeling of being terribly different was so great that he could never feel contact or contacted. Jasper exploited his conviction (that difference makes understanding impossible) in such a way as to avoid actually confronting his fears that he would never be recognized because of his difference. In our relationship, an intimation of sameness or overlapping experience or mutuality was skipped over and ignored because hiding behind that false promise of complete understanding lurked the terrible shock of difference that feels irreconcilable. It was so persuasive that it took all of our energy to avoid seeing it. I agreed, for a while, to terminating in order to avoid seeing it, until I was able to turn my attention back to the task of analyzing.

Once we agreed to continue our work, the problem of the meanings of difference became a central organizing question for both of us. One way to understand my feeling, that an obvious overlap of experience that existed between the two of us had been ignored and denied, was that it was just this kind of misattunement that had dominated important relationships in Jasper's life and led to a pervasive sense of going unrecognized. Perhaps I had to carry these disavowed feelings of going unrecognized in our relationship, until we found a way to enable Jasper to recover the experiences that he could not contain.

As Aron (1996) has so effectively described, the analytic encounter is asymmetric, but it can be mutual when an understanding that each party's subjectivity is crucial to the analysis is made explicit. The asymmetry, due to the analyst's abstemious conscious expression of subjectivity, guarantees the ongoing study of the analysand's subjective experience in the work. My disclosure of my serostatus to Jasper no doubt complicated our relationship. But through and with these complications we were able to move toward analyzing material that felt inaccessible to me and full of danger to Jasper. I contaminated the transference, but the transference was being avoided in order to avoid contamination. Perhaps we required some kind of contamination in order to move into the transference in greater detail.

What if the transference is not contaminated with this particular disclosure? When the serostatus of the analyst is revealed after symptoms are observable, the question from the analysand's point of view might be, "How could you have conducted my analysis while keeping this from me?" Conversely, in the event that the analyst reveals seropositivity to the analysand before any apparent physical change, the question might be, "How can you expect me to continue in treatment while knowing this about you?" Both, I believe, are analyzable situations. But what are the criteria through which one option is preferred to the other? To a certain extent, the avoidance of disclosure, of admitting contagion into the room, has to do with the privileged place of autonomy as an overarching value in psychoanalytic culture. Kohut (1971) mounted an important critique of this privileging of autonomy and independence at the expense of vital and vitalizing dependency throughout one's life, but his technique, strictly practiced, doesn't allow for a condition or need of the analyst to become an explicit part of the process. My seropositivity brought into sharp detail how the autonomy and independence of the analyst are maintained and how one disguises the other in our theories of technique.

What would it be like to say to a patient, "I can work with you, but I need you to know something about me because it has potential impact on our work together?" This might be experienced as seductive, demanding, burdensome. Or it might be experienced as open, vulnerable, and intimate. Or both. The statement contains an expression of need on the part of the analyst and so seems to undermine the analyst's neutrality, but also, and perhaps more threatening, the analyst's autonomy. It is a direct refutation of the fantasy that the analyst is detached, free of desire for the patient.

One day, as Jasper and I were talking about the "messy, juicy" parts of his psychic life that he was leaving out of our interactions, he asked if I was saying that I required him to talk about this material. I responded that I didn't think of my position as one that required anything from him, that it was up to him to determine what was accomplished in our work. I added that I did wish he would tell me what we had noticed he was avoiding. At first I had hesitated to answer his question; I wondered if I ought to put my response solely in terms of what would be most useful to his treatment. But doing this seemed inadequate to me. What I experienced was desire, and I felt it was important to express this. Unspoken desire, present in every treatment, was keeping us both inside that car. Jasper's conviction was that the overwhelming desires he contained could never be comprehensible, let alone acceptable, to another. But it seemed to me at this point that at least my desire could be articulated—my desire to know more, to know that which he was convinced was unacceptable and unknowable.

Through this ironic twist, it was I who ended up in the position of wanting to know and of feeling left out. Jasper had repeatedly told me that he tried not to have questions about me. At the point when I disclosed my serostatus to him, it was clear that he was doing his utmost not to know this about me. Here he turned around the question that analysts pose regarding disclosure: "Does the patient genuinely want to know?" I found myself answering him that I did genuinely want to know. After that moment, we attended to the meanings of Jasper's determination not to have questions about me, and his way of managing himself. The specific relational style that Jasper uses to avoid contact was obviously an important area for us to investigate, but we also saw the way that we distracted ourselves from confronting the question about whether the patient really wishes to know. It was as if having technique provides the rationale for avoiding this question. So long as we can remain focused on a technique, so long as we remain convinced that the question the patient is really wanting to ask and not to ask is about, say, desire and the primal scene, we can avoid considering the question whether the patient really wants to know anything about us.

I certainly did not intend to disclose any further information about myself to Jasper, though it is easy to imagine that I could have. But I am skeptical of the implications of the position I occupy as the arbiter of what the patient genuinely wishes to know. Often I need to advocate for a patient's multiplicity, for his complicatedness in the face of a wish to see himself as transparent and simple.

But to avoid asking and answering what the patient really wishes to know puts me in the uncomfortably omnipotent position of a kind of gatekeeper of another's subjectivity. This seems to me the opposite of the job I assume when I offer myself as someone to whom a patient can tell anything. The job is about opening the gate and believing in the potential that it can remain open to traffic in both directions.

Jasper and I did agree on a termination date, in three and one-half years. As the time grew nearer to our final session, Jasper told me:

> "The pivotal moment was around the time of your companion's death and those sessions after, when I found out you were HIV positive. Because for a while it seemed as if I was going to have to make your needs more important than mine. And I found out that that wasn't going to happen. The men I have always wanted to be close to—my father—never wanted me. But you encouraged it. I had to keep you out of it. Right now I'm noticing that I'm feeling as if you're an equal—that we're talking peer to peer instead of a needy little boy talking to the all-powerful father who's not going to want me. I guess I lose that . . . that feeling like I need to be taken care of, that I'm not able to take care of myself."

In the termination phase we both understood that Jasper had transformed the way he experienced himself, with the requisite mourning the loss of the dependent little boy that such a shift always entails. Desire of another kind, between peers, was acknowledged, safely. Jasper had gotten out of the car.

CHAPTER 4

A Duty to Disclose?

FOUR YEARS AFTER THE OBITUARY of my late partner prompted the disclosures to Kent and Jasper, the question of disclosing my HIV status in the initial consultation arose when I met Jack. A sophisticated young man, well spoken and obviously intelligent, he described his previous experiences in psychotherapy:

"My first therapist was an analyst. She was brilliant, I think, and although I wasn't seeking out an analysis, I soon found myself going to her three times a week and lying on the couch. It all came tumbling out, and it was clear that I had really needed this kind of experience. I do believe that it was transformative. Then we were about two and a half years into it, and she told me that she was going on a two-week vacation. Well, I didn't know it then, and I didn't find out for a very long time after, but she really was going into the hospital for major surgery. Apparently something went wrong on the table, and she was incapacitated for months. I never heard about what had happened. When the two weeks passed, I went for my appointment, and she wasn't there. There was no word about her, no nothing. I later learned that she did, in fact, recover enough to give her friends and colleagues the impression that she had called her patients, but she hadn't. Finally, she did eventually start to practice again, and I saw her, but it was clear to me that something was wrong. I saw her two or three times and then decided to stop. Six months after that, I learned that she had died.

It was only at the memorial service that I learned what had actually happened, and that by the time I was with her, she had only a very few patients. A couple of years later, a friend who knew what had happened pointed out an article about your analyst dying while you're in analysis. As I read it, it dawned on me that this was written by another one of my former analyst's patients. I sort of went into a meltdown right then. Cried for about two hours . . .

Eventually, I realized that I needed to work out some things about what had happened, and I interviewed several therapists and finally decided on this one. But after working with her for three months or so, I felt as if I was not being managed very well. She was very warm but, somehow, not professional or, well, seasoned. I left that treatment . . .

What I'm looking for now is not necessarily about working through what happened with my first analyst, because I feel as if I have done that. I want to feel that what I'm doing with my life is not just filling the time. That's what it feels like I'm doing, simply finding ways of filling the days, as if I'm drifting. I'm having a good time, but nothing really feels very . . . important.

This consultation presented me with a dilemma. It seemed to me that basic clinical practices regarding disclosure, abstinence, and neutrality were tangled up with certain ethical questions.

In his 1915 paper, "Further recommendations in the technique of psycho-analysis: Observations on transference love," Freud is unequivocal: "psycho-analytic treatment is founded on truthfulness. In this fact lies a great part of its educative effect and its ethical value" (p. 164). Three themes are introduced in this statement: truthfulness, educative effects, and ethical values. As I listened to Jack describe the mysterious events surrounding the death of his former analyst, the themes of my own truthfulness and my ethical stance pressed in on me, demanding to be rethought. I was confronted with an imperative duty to tell a prospective patient that I am HIV positive.

In the many years that I have practiced with this knowledge of myself, this question has occurred to me in various contexts. Each time it felt possible to put off actually making the disclosure for such reasons as deciding that a disclosure of this kind would burden the patient or that I might be colluding with the patient's ambivalence about entering treatment, or because a prospective patient seemed so narcissistically vulnerable that he would not be interested in me as another human subjectivity. These are *clinical* reasons not to disclose personal medical information.

Handling clinical situations such as those I've mentioned is addressed in recommendations on technique, which are based on theories of psychic functioning and therapeutic action. Freud's (1912) advice on technique is multitextured. As I've pointed out, he states that he values truthfulness above all. He also frankly describes his recommendations as formulated through his frustrating experiences with patients. Apparently he tried other approaches, but he cautions other analysts to refrain from making disclosures of personal information, recommending instead that the analyst maintain an opaque, or mirror-like reserve.

With time, this technical stance became understood as one aspect of how the analyst establishes and protects the analytic frame, a boundary around the treatment relationship. The analytic frame refers also to the consistent time and frequency of sessions and such issues as foregoing contact beyond the analytic hour. This boundedness yields therapeutic benefits, which are theorized in a particular way within each of three broadly defined models of psychoanalytic therapeutic action (Mitchell, 1988a): drive conflict, developmental arrest, and relational conflict.

THE ANALYTIC FRAME AND THEORIES OF THERAPEUTIC ACTION

In the drive-conflict model, the analytic frame works to unveil and magnify the reemergence of the infantile wishes and fantasies. By refraining from informing the patient of any personal information, the analyst theoretically remains anonymous, so as to allow the patient to experience the analyst as fully as possible as an old object in the reworking of these unremembered but lived conflicts of early life. The technical advice to remain anonymous, to maintain the distinct analytic frame, is consonant with a theory of mind that regards motivation as emanating from biologically determined drives and the difficulties of forming appropriate compromise formations so as to achieve adequate drive satisfaction. This is a one-mind theory of therapeutic action. The anonymous analyst offers himself or herself as a screen for the replaying of unremembered conflicts. Any contributions from the analyst other than interpretations of resistance to remembering are, at best, superfluous, and generally regarded as unfortunate examples of the analyst's inability to allow the process to unfold in its natural course.

In the developmental-arrest model, a patient's difficulties are the result of failure on the part of primary caregivers to provide adequate emotional supplies that enable the person to consolidate a cohesive, organized, and robust self-structure. The development of the self (Kohut, 1971) or the emergence of the true self (Winnicott, 1960) are theorized as primary motivations for human beings, and problems in self-development are the basic examples of psychopathology. Difficulties that appear to resemble pathologies of conflict are secondary to flaws in the self-structure. Therapeutic action, therefore, is oriented toward permitting the self to resume its natural development through—for example, in Kohutian self psychology—the provision of the idealizing and mirroring that, it is posited, are required for optimal development of a cohesive self. The analyst, through empathy, attempts to understand the patient's experience from the patient's point of view, and to convey this understanding. The analyst demonstrates the capacity to provide the mirroring and idealization the patient requires to promote the consolidation of the faulty self-structure. The analytic frame works to orient the analyst in this endeavor, particularly through the inevitable failures of empathy. The analyst is conceptualized in this model as a new object, one that is unencumbered by his or her own needs or conflicts. The analytic frame assists the analyst in this presentation.

Frequently, however, the maintenance of the frame itself is experienced by the patient as a failure of empathy. Such matters as regular sessions, no extra-session contacts, and payment of the fee can feel to a patient whose self-structure is exceptionally fragile as further examples of a world that is hostile to what seem like basic needs. As in the drive-conflict model, the maintenance of the analytic frame works to keep the analyst's contributions to a minimum. In the developmental-arrest model, though, therapeutic action occurs through the exquisite attention to and repair of the inevitable failures of empathy. It is the repair of these empathic breaches that promotes maturation, what Kohut termed "transmuting internalizations" (1971, p. 28). Once again, this is a one-mind model, and so the analytic frame is integrally connected with how the mind is theorized to function, and how therapy is theorized to cure (Kohut, 1984).

The third model, relational conflict, offers the most potential flexibility in terms of what is meant by maintaining the analytic frame. For an analyst working in this theoretical mode, the relationship to the frame may be the most open to negotiation, which brings potential benefits as well as certain risks. In this model, the mind is theorized as developing in and through the determining context of the web of relationships throughout an individual's life. The subject is an active organizer of his experience; the distinctive style of that organization is one manifestation of a personal idiom (Bollas, 1987). Enduring relational styles, including those that seem problematic, are theorized to produce a sense of equilibrium, as the person can predict and ensure the provision of required emotional supplies. Psychopathology is identified to the extent to which the individual's relational system is open or closed: whether new experience can be integrated or is shunned in favor of repetition of old patterns. Primary motivation is the establishment of the particular quality of connection with others. Relationships are basic. Therapeutic action, in this model, involves the analyst's entrance into the patient's relational patterns, which the patient is unconsciously compelled to repeat with the analyst. The analyst's contributions, determined by his or her own idiosyncratic ways of relating, make up half of this relationship. It is through the living out of the relational pattern and the retrospective analysis of the enactments in which the analyst and patient engage each other, that insight and change occur. (For contemporary views of enactments as the living out of unconscious or dissociated relational patterns in the treatment relationship, see Bromberg, 1998, and Hoffman, 1998.) The analyst can be experienced as a new object via the working through of the old pattern, and a relatively closed relational system can be opened up through this process.

In this model, then, the analytic frame might be seen as the most potentially porous, in that the understanding of the anonymity of the analyst is so different. In the relational-conflict model, the frame might be thought of as a point of orientation, rather than as an ideal the analyst seeks to maintain. Purposeful disclosures of personal data would not be regarded as necessary for living out the enactments that comprise the action of therapy. But neither would such disclosures be regarded as destructive to the treatment, insofar as *any* contributions from the analyst to the ongoing process are potentially useful. The salient question in the relational-conflict model is not whether to make a particular disclosure—or, once one is (inadvertently or otherwise) made, how to correct this mistake—but what is the best use that can be made of a disclosure (Ehrenberg, 1995; Greenberg, 1995).

The most dramatic transgressions of the frame (that is, engaging in a sexual relationship with a patient) are discussed primarily in terms of a breakthrough of unmanageable countertransference feelings, and secondarily as ethical breaches. In such examples, it is sometimes argued that the relatively authoritative and powerful position that the analyst occupies, in contrast to the relative dependence and neediness of the patient, has been exploited so that the analyst's responses to a patient's material, as well as the unconscious and unanalyzed needs of the analyst, take precedence over the well-being of the patient. Often such breaches are described as the outcome of an accumulation of lesser violations of the analytic frame; the analyst, all too late, finds that he or she has slid down a slippery slope (Davies, 2000). In this context, then, the analytic frame functions as the guardian against the analyst's unruly erotic wishes.

One of the results of this way of focusing on erotic acting out is that transgression and vulnerability are combined, with the unfortunate effect that the analyst's vulnerability may not be given sufficient attention.

A tremendous distance exists between the traditional role of the analyst that is reflected in early analytic literature and the contemporary analyst who has emerged "from behind the wizard's curtain [with] . . . the general acceptance of the shift from a 'one-person' to a 'two-person' psychology" (Pizer, 2000, p. 197). Psychoanalysts continue to struggle with the dissonance emerging between the construction of the psychoanalyst in our theory and literature that describes an idealized maturity, austerity, and restraint that sometimes pushes the analyst's capacity to a breaking point, and our experience of ourselves as ordinary, vulnerable human beings. Although contemporary analysts may wish to come out from behind the wizard's curtain, our patients' dynamics (as well as our own dynamics such as idealization of the role of analyst) and responses to our vulnerabilities complicate our coming out.

Indeed, the situation in which I found myself with Jack, a dilemma that felt to me not exhaustively a *clinical* one, but also an ethical one, required a rethinking of my relationship not only to the analytic frame, but also to certain idealizations posited and supported in psychoanalytic theory and literature. It became necessary to examine an experience of vulnerability, not only in a private sphere, but also in relation to patients and prospective patients. In this case, relying on the recommendations with regard to maintaining the analytic frame helped me insofar as my feelings of vulnerability and powerlessness could remain hidden. Do the technical recommendations function as a taboo against speaking of vulnerability, dependence, illness, and death in such a way as to obscure these issues from our own awareness?

The recent critique of power relations in the analytic situation, inspired by Fouacult (e.g., Dimen, 1995), has tended to speak only of the power held by the analyst over patients. Rarely do analysts openly consider the power that their patients (or, in my case, potential patients) have over them. Certainly we do occupy positions of relative power. People come to analysts hoping to get help. The analytic frame and other recommendations regarding technique are important guidelines that provide clinical leverage as well as protection for a patient from potential exploitation. It is unarguable that the partners in any analytic situation are not equals, but they are not equal in different ways. Analysts need patients to analyze, not only because our financial security depends on it, but also because our self-esteem does. To be able to work with patients who can use our skill to bring more freedom and creativity into their own lives is a wonderful experience. We devote extensive periods of time to training, ongoing study, and consultation in order to do this. But we depend on our patients for the opportunity to put our work into practice. What I hope to make explicit is the question of how the analyst's dependence and vulnerability are hidden by certain technical practices.

Countertransference and the Ethical Ground

On this occasion I found that I did not wish to refrain from making a disclosure. Jack's real experience of losing his valued analyst (and more important, the silence and obfuscation around that experience) led me to feel that it was imperative that I depart from the relative comfort of remaining silent. Although I operate assuming that I will survive the length of any new treatment that I take on, I could not offer my services without making Jack aware of the potential of my becoming ill because of a condition I did know about when he began analysis. Knowing also that I cannot expect to *guarantee* him that I will survive for as long as we work together (a guarantee that no one really can make), I did know that I *could* guarantee him that his experience of losing an analyst and not knowing anything about the circumstances of that loss would not be repeated. Beginning with the familiar process of attempting to analyze the countertransference, I understood this question's urgent quality to be associated with identifications I felt with both Jack and his former analyst. Perhaps I wished, in a rather omnipotent way, to avoid a repetition of experiences of illness, mystification, and loss, in his life and in my own. It was important to note how the interpenetrations of my own experiences of loss, my fears of potential illness, were implicated in this sense of urgency.

The urgency emphasized the atmosphere of constraint, almost taboo, when it came to speaking of illness and death. Certainly, Jack's attitude was rather diffident on the matter of working through the loss of his former analyst. I did not feel that it was appropriate in the initial interview to press him on this. But I was acutely aware of two dynamics that dominated my experience of the meeting with Jack: my desire, and the death of analysts. It is noteworthy that the cultural construction of HIV/AIDS that lingers still is the conjunction of desire and death. Psychoanalysis from its inception sought to overcome the taboo of speaking openly of sexuality, a battle that, in some obvious respects, has been won. And in some ways, the societal response to HIV/AIDS reveals how sexuality continues to arouse unconscious terrors that have deleterious material effects. Our psychoanalytic cultural tradition of speaking frankly of sex is built on the conviction that this is therapeutic. One way of understanding what I felt at this point was the stronger taboo of speaking of the other element that comprises how HIV/AIDS is represented: in the case of Jack and me, the analyst's illness and death.

However, in that initial consultation, I did not speak up. The clamor of interior voices arguing for and against disclosure was too much for me in that session, and anyway I couldn't be sure that Jack was really interested in working with me. Perhaps he'd choose someone else, and I'd be off the hook.

That was not to be. The next day he called to tell me that he'd like to begin work, and to schedule regular appointments. This we did quickly, and as I hung up the phone, I realized that I felt as if I couldn't begin work with this man without scheduling another consultation in which he could learn something about me that I felt would affect his decision about whom he'd choose as his therapist. As I moved toward this realization, as I rehearsed my pitch and talked it over with colleagues, I felt, more fully than at any other time, my fear of being rejected because I am HIV positive. My hands shook. My stomach turned over. When I made the phone call to request this additional consultation, my voice quavered. Jack asked why I was making this request, and it was all I could do not to stammer. I said that I did not wish to be mysterious, but that there was some information about me that I felt was important to share with him before making a decision about working together. He agreed to come in, and we found a time.

On the morning of the appointment, that wave of anxiety swept over me again. When he came into my office, I cut to the chase. I thanked him for making the time for this additional appointment, and then said that I wished to tell him was that I am HIV positive. I added that, having heard about his previous experience, it seemed impossible to begin work with him without telling him about this.

Without missing a beat, Jack responded that this in no way affected his decision, and that he was grateful that I'd told him. He asked if I tell all of my patients about my seropositivity?

Now that I'd begun to tell him about myself, could I stop? "Well," I replied, "no. I am in process on this and do not have a consistent policy about telling patients. Maybe I *should* tell everyone I work with. I was certain that I could not begin with you without telling. So, what is this like for you?"

"Well, as odd as it may seem, AIDS has not affected me directly. Not at all. That may surprise you, because I am the only gay man my age I know who has not been directly affected by it. Well, I have dated guys who were HIV positive, and I must have had sex with guys who were. But it never seemed to be an issue. Safe sex was never a problem since I came out so late, after AIDS was on the scene and we knew the importance of safe sex. And I haven't been in the position of taking care of anyone who's been ill. So, it really hasn't touched my life at all."

"So perhaps my telling you about my HIV status feels like an irrelevant intrusion?"

"No, I fully understand why you have told me, and I appreciate it. I don't really have much else to say. I came in a listening mode today, I guess."

With a few more exchanges, the consultation ended, not having taken up the whole hour. Jack wished to return to work. I was relieved, confused, tired.

I had been aware that Jack appealed to me as a patient when

we first met. He described what is to me a very good reason to enter psychoanalytic treatment: to develop a greater sense of meaning in life. So I was extremely happy that he'd chosen me. In time, I allowed other feelings to register. I was thunderstruck that he'd told me that HIV/AIDS had not affected his life at all, thunderstruck and resentful. So, could I have made this disclosure with a retaliatory motive? I worried that a retaliation might have been disguised in the way that, in this extra consultation, the initial establishment of the frame, which included this particular disclosure, might be destructive to the treatment. Further, I felt guilty about my relief that the extra consultation had lasted only a half session, noting that I had not maintained even the basic frame of a fifty-minute treatment hour. As I went over this moment, I was struck by the rather breezy way Jack set aside not only HIV/AIDS, but also his lived experiences of illness and loss.

For gay men of my generation, HIV/AIDS was, for a very long time, the ubiquitous ground for our lives, even with the newer generations of medications that, for many, forestall the opportunistic infections that dominated the experience of the seropositive person in the 1980s and early 1990s. The social context for the disclosure of HIV status, then, has a vast array of different meanings. A traditional psychoanalyst might understand this solely as a display due to my inability to withstand the abstemiousness required of the analyst. In the literature on the analyst's illness, Wong (cited in Schwartz and Silver, 1990) suggested that a disclosure of being sick could be understood as narcissistic exhibitionism. I wish to counter, or to augment, that interpretation by pointing out that, partly to work against the awful memories and fears of AIDS and partly as an indication of the integration of HIV/AIDS as a manageable chronic condition, the disclosure of HIV seropositivity is a highly overdetermined statement. Without seeking to minimize the multiplicity of meaning involved in any disclosure, a leading edge of my conscious reasons for telling Jack this was the importance of being honest about a fact of my life that had the potential to affect an open-ended treatment relationship.

Clearly, this is not a sufficient description of the disclosure, but it is also not a negligible one. The literature on disclosure in psychoanalysis distinguishes between telling a patient personal data and revealing emotional responses to the patient. At this juncture with Jack, it seems that I was straddling, somehow, this differentiation. What was possible to regard as a piece of personal data was also drenched in possible meanings, to me and to Jack. Perhaps what I was honest about, then, when I told Jack about my status, was that I would not be trying to control the field of meaning-making between the two of us, but would make explicit what might be a part of what determines how I make meaning.

A compelling aspect of the analytic situation, defined to a degree by the frame, is that analysts sometimes describe feeling more themselves during the work than at other times, or being a better version of themselves (Schafer, 1983). There is a wonderful paradox operating here: in a situation where, generally, personal data remains unreported, as well as some but certainly not all of the analyst's emotional responses to the patient, working within these constraints still yields an experience of being more genuine. That sense of the genuine emerges from an experience of connection, interpenetration, and unveiling. A growing body of contemporary literature seems preoccupied with this theme of maintaining and expressing the analyst's genuine presence within the frame. My own concerns with establishing a genuine presence contributed to my desire to disclose, to deviate from the frame, as well.

In this initial meeting with Jack, I confronted quite vividly my desires with regard to a new patient. Understandable desire to gain an insightful new patient, desire to enable him to have a different kind of experience from his previous one with an analyst, and perhaps unconscious desires to enact something about illness and loss through and with this patient. These latter desires were one subject of my ongoing reflection as the treatment unfolded. Thinking over the first moments with this patient, I can now be sure that the awareness of my desire that Jack would choose me did put me on guard. Prior to meeting with him, I was more confidently convinced about *clinical* reasons not to inform prospective patients of a fact that was, and remains, only a potential disruption to a treatment undertaken with me. All along, I was also aware of a feeling of relief when such rationalizations for not disclosing assured me that remaining silent was appropriate. I became strongly aware of my sense of power-lessness in the situation, my vulnerability, because I was convinced that anyone knowing of my status would no longer see me as a viable analyst and elect not to work with me.

So, gauging these feelings, I was alerted to an immediate response to Jack that in some way interacted with my anxieties about a genuine presence, honesty, and possibly my ethical duty to present reasons that might dissuade him from choosing me. The fantasy that this attractive, successful man would be engaged in analytic work with me, and that he would pass my name along to acquaintances in his fashionable, successful crowd, was quick to blossom. It is a fantasy that embarrasses me to admit. But as Jack took on these meanings in my imagination, the stakes concerning his choosing me got higher. And accordingly, so did my anxiety about admitting to my infected state.

Some months after we began treatment, Jack revealed his awareness of a rather dismissive attitude toward me. I asked him how this came to his attention. He recalled the time he told me that he found the way I dressed "quaintly amusing" (in cooler weather I usually wear corduroy pants and plaid flannel shirts) and another occasion when he casually mentioned that he was certain he made far more money than I did. He said he imagined that he did this to counteract the feelings of attraction he had toward me. He'd told his best friend that he wondered whether I'd be a good therapist for him because he'd found me so attractive in our first consultation. His friend argued, Jack told me, that this was precisely the best reason to choose me, because Jack wanted therapy to help him establish an enduring romantic relationship. For my part, learning that he'd been attracted to me but wished not to tell me confirmed my sense that aspects of desire and loss had consciously been set aside from discussion. I found a new reason for worry: that I had colluded with his avoidance of the most painful matters by telling him I was HIV-positive in an attempt to counter his attraction. It also struck me that our interaction repeated a negotiation that occurs between potential lovers when they first meet, an event that is now commonplace. It is also a negotiation whose genuineness depends on the honesty of the partners.

Analyzing the countertransference felt like much more familiar territory than teasing out the ethical considerations that pertain to this instance of beginning a new treatment. Indeed, any consideration of the analyst's vulnerability has been, by definition, an analysis of countertransference. But the interaction between our private experience, possibly and in varying degrees overlapping with what we think of as countertransference, and professional ideals is not always obvious. Further complicating matters is what I think of as a transference to the field of psychoanalysis itself, where a body of technique has been proposed and theorized. One of the effects that a theory of technique may have is to obscure the philosophical and ethical subtext, what we might think of as a latent content of a psychoanalytic consciousness.

THINKING THROUGH THE DILEMMA

In a retrospective attempt to regain my bearings, I reviewed the ethics standards set by some of the professional organizations to which analysts belong. I then scanned the work of major exemplars of ethical concepts in order to understand the elaboration or disguises of ethical themes in psychoanalytic literature on theory and practice. In setting out to find assistance in thinking through my own situation, what I confronted is that analytic theory and technical advice obscure questions of the analyst's vulnerability in relation to patients, and lead, in some cases, to positions that are ethically uncomfortable for the analyst.

ESTABLISHED CODES OF ETHICS

Because psychoanalysis began as a medical specialty, beginning was easy: with the Hippocratic Oath, specifically the directive, "First, do no harm." Our primary responsibility is to those who have entrusted us with their care. At this first step, we encounter the question of whether withholding personal information could be interpreted as potentially doing harm. But how have our responsibilities been further elaborated? The *Ethical Principles of Psychologists and Code of Conduct* (American Psychological Association, 1992) and the *Code of Ethics of the Clinical Social Work Federation* (1997) set forth tenets that arguably but only implicitly touch on the situation in which I find myself. Principle B of the psychologists' *Code of Conduct* states that "Psychologists seek to promote integrity" (p. 6). In the first article of the social work *Code of Ethics*, we are told that "clinical social workers . . . value professional competence, objectivity, and integrity. . . . They accept responsibility for the consequences of their work (p. 2)." How exactly is the ideal integrity operationalized? Psychologists "are honest, fair, and respectful of others. . . . [They] do not make statements that are false, misleading, or deceptive. . . . [they] strive to be aware of their own belief systems, values, needs, and limitations and the effect of these on their work. . . . Psychologists avoid improper and potentially harmful dual relationships" (1992, p. 6). Social workers, according their code, "do not exploit professional relationships sexually, financially or for any other professional and/or personal advantage" (1997, p. 2).

Psychoanalytically trained clinicians may already sense the complicated quality of these proscriptions. In my case, for example, how confident can I be that agreeing to work with anyone in open-ended psychoanalytically oriented therapy does not include an element of exploitation in the sense both of my financial dependence on patients and my interest in bolstering my own experience of ongoing competence, vitality, and independence?

Principle D of the psychologists' code affirms their respect for all persons' self-determination (1992, p. 7). Article II of the social work code states that clinical social workers "maximize the self-determination of the clients with whom they work" (p. 3). To what, exactly, does the phrase self-determination refer? It is obvious that a prospective analysand has the right to choose us or not, but to maximize the self-determination of this choice, can it be argued that it is thus incumbent on us to reveal details of our private lives such as the state of our health?

In section 3 of this article of the social work code, on "relationships with clients," we are enjoined to set "appropriate boundaries" (p. 5). Special emphasis is given to those situations in which a clinician may be working with persons who are related to each other. Romantic and sexual relationships with clients are prohibited. Therapists are enjoined not to abuse the authority inherent in the professional role. Again the right to self-determination is invoked, with regard to the problems of confidentiality and insurance companies. Finally, when a conflict "potentially detrimental to the treatment" arises, a clinical social worker has the duty to inform the client (p. 6). The *Code of Ethics of the National Association of Social Workers* (1996) does not differ in content from these articles. It adds: "In some cases, protecting clients' interests may require termination of the professional relationship with proper referral of the client" (p. 9).

The potential conflict between the importance of appropriate boundaries and such values as self-determination and what may be potentially detrimental to the treatment process is necessarily unspecified. There is no way to specify the infinite number of possible scenarios in which these values might clash. Already, there is a tangle of competing ideals here. For example, in the interest of maintaining appropriate boundaries, we might decide to refrain from making disclosures of any kind, given the possibility of the seductive dynamic inherent in sharing personal information. However, increasing the self-determination and autonomy of a prospective client might lead us to feel the need to selectively disclose personal information. The ethical codes governing a professional group such as social workers seem potentially to conflict with the specialized subgroup of psychoanalysts who are, as in my case, social workers.

The *Guides on Professional Conduct for Psychoanalysts* (Michaels, 1969), countering the "unspoken" requirements for the conduct of psychoanalysts (p. 294) that echoed Freud's remark that "as to morals, that goes without saying" (Freud, S. 1905b, p. 267), record the efforts to achieve a code of ethics for the American Psychoanalytic Association. One of the difficulties that Michaels specifies is the potentially conflicting loyalties with which the psychoanalyst contends: "to his community, to his profession at large (physicians), to his speciality with its specific conditions, to his colleagues and contemporaries, to his professional institution, to his medical school or teaching hospital, to his students, whom he analyses or supervises, and last, but not least, to his patients" (p. 299).

Most of the ethical considerations in Michaels's recommendations are financial. The category that most nearly addresses the matter of the analyst's medical condition and the relationship with patients is "Transference and Countertransference: . . . any misconception by the analyst leading to his personal and emotional involvement will be avoided. "If the analyst, in a special situation, cannot master his countertransference by self-analysis or through an additional analysis of his acute difficulty, he should transfer that case to another analyst" (Michaels, 1969, p. 304). Special situations, a term so broad as to encompass all that cannot be anticipated, are dispatched when they become too unruly by referring the case to another analyst. What is taken very seriously into consideration, and rightly so, is the vulnerability of the patient. Should the analyst be tempted to reveal vulnerability of her or his own, this would be considered an abuse of the transference/countertransference relationship. The analyst's condition as a subject requiring ethical consideration disappears, covered over by the ethical code predicated on a theory of therapeutic action, based in turn on a theory of how the mind works.

The final draft of the *Proposed Revision of Principles and Standards of Ethics for Psychoanalysis*, dated January 16, 2001, from the American Psychoanalytic Association, pointedly takes into account the complexities of the analytic situation. Rather than defining what ethical behavior is, analysts are expected to reflect and to seek consultation when the most ethical way of confronting a difficult situation is not obvious (pp. 1–2). The 2001 revision is in this way consonant with recent theoretical elaboration. For example, the development of the two-person, relational, or intersubjective models of the psychoanalytic situation (and of mental functioning in general), the once transparent concept of appropriate boundaries, has become rather cloudy. Disclosure of subjective responses to the analysand, including erotic feelings (e.g., Davies, 1994), is becoming more openly discussed.

The question of making such disclosures is most often debated in the context of clinical utility and therapeutic action. The ethical dimension, to the extent that it is made explicit, often has to do with dismantling the power differential between analyst and analysand, where it is assumed, accurately so, that the analyst occupies the position of power. But the matter of the analyst's vulnerability seems far more difficult to consider. This is a problem that has occupied psychoanalysts from the earliest days of the psychoanalytic movement, the best example being Ferenczi's contributions, which have recently enjoyed renewed interest. In his experiments with mutual analysis, and in "Confusion of Tongues" (Ferenczi, 1933), he explicitly tested power relations as well as the traditional frame in the analytic situation. That he was expelled from the psychoanalytic establishment and his contributions discredited toward the end of his life demonstrate vividly the hostility directed at an analyst who challenged the dominant rules of technique and theory, and who thought independently. It is also a poignant illustration of the vulnerability of the analyst who dares to do so.

THE CLASSICAL TRADITION AND ETHICAL TRANSPARENCY

Freud had little to say on the subject of ethics with regard specifically to the practice of psychoanalysis: "I consider ethics to be taken for granted. Actually I have never done a mean thing" (quoted in Jones, 1957, p. 247).

Freud's seminal work with hysterics in Victorian-era Vienna was, in a crucial way, guided by an ethical goal: to uncover the sexual hypocrisy of a prevailing social order that, in his estimation, caused the suffering of his patients. So from the very earliest days of the psychoanalytic movement, ethics has been conflated with psychic phenomena. Freud strove to demonstrate that psychoanalysis is an empirically valid science that requires that the analyst's contribution be separable from the analytic situation. Thus, whatever personal events or difficulties the analyst contends with will have been resolved in a training analysis, or, if necessary, could be addressed in a return to analysis. This isolated-mind model of psychoanalytic work owes most of its construction to the ideals of empirical science, and in turn the explicit ethical codes for analyst's behavior are arguably influenced by the ideals this model holds out to us. And because psychoanalysis is a professional practice in which the analyst occupies a position of relative power, it is appropriate that the primary considerations when we approach ethical dilemmas are clinical. But the situation in which I found myself with Jack, feeling pressed by the knowledge of how he lost his previous analyst and my serostatus, leads me to the conviction that this is only a partial description. Perhaps owing to my strong identification with psychoanalysis, I surveyed a sampling of classical analytic literature that takes up ethics in an attempt to think through the question of the analyst's disappearing vulnerability.

The classical literature regarding ethics or morality often describes how psychoanalytic treatment leads to the development of higher order ethical beliefs and behaviors in the analysand (Levy-Suhl, 1946; Money-Kyrle, 1952; Hartmann, 1960; Nielsen, 1960). In these works elaborating how the development of a personal ethics takes place, it is possible to discern two sharply contrasting ethical systems dominating the conversation. The clash between these philosophies was an important part of the intellectual world of Freud's student days (Gay, 1990). One is the universal ethics of Kant (1785) principally expressed in his "Categorical Imperative." The other is the writing of Nietzsche (1887), who, disagreeing sharply with Kant, argued for a personal approach to ethics that privileged truth, cut though what he regarded as hypocrisy, and is perhaps best expressed in his concept of the "eternal return of the same" (p. 273). Kant's transcendentalist analysis and Nietzsche's vigorous antitranscendentalist response are each discernable in samples of psychoanalytic literature, as well as in the construction of the ethical role of the analyst. Before arguing that these philosophers' ideas can be found in how analysts have written about their clinical work, the contrast between Kant's and Nietzsche's ideas must be made clear.

To make that contrast most vivid requires a highly simplified and schematic presentation of these philosophers' thought. We also must break into a conversation that was long underway. Kant, answering Descartes's radical doubt about how we come to know about the existence of anything, wanted to move from a "popular moral philosophy," which is vulnerable to situational and personal variation, to a "metaphysics of morals," which set forth permanent, universal rules. The clearest description of this universal rule, one that Kant conceived in order to transcend the relativity inherent in a conception of personal moral code, is his Categorical Imperative.

Kant's (1785) Imperative is formulated in several ways. In the first, supreme principle of morality, he posits that we must always act in such a way that we would want the rules guiding our individual actions to become universal laws. Another formulation of the Imperative states that we should always treat all people as ends in themselves and never as means to an end. This injunction works also for the actor as well; we must treat ourselves as ends, and never a means to an end. Kant's aim in composing the Imperative was to provide a reliable formula for consistent ethical behavior, one that would be free of the potential for lapses owing to individuals' competing needs and abuses of power.

Arguments criticizing Kant's Categorical Imperative have asserted that he offers only an empty formula of little use in devising specific rules that can guide human behavior in actual lived situations. But perhaps it is just this lack of specific content that is precisely its strength. Certainly the values Kant expressed are apparent in the constitutions of modern democracies, as well as in the Golden Rule. But for Kant's Imperative to be effective, the person must be strongly identified with the universal to achieve a higher order of ethical life. At the very least, the Imperative requires that every act be seriously considered before being carried out, thus demanding a particular kind of relationship between the person and the world.

Although Freud denied reading any but a fragment of Nietzsche's work, his popularity among circles Freud was likely to frequent, during his student days as well as when he was building the psychoanalytic movement, has made some skeptical of Freud's protest (Lehrer, 1995). Relevant to the development of psychoanalytic thought is the recognition that Nietzsche, like Freud, was reacting against what he felt was a vast tradition of hypocrisy about what motivates human behavior. Nietzsche (1887) was highly skeptical of the notion of an ordinary person's capacity for identification with an ideal such as Kant's Universal. He referred to what appeared to be altruistic motives with particular contempt, arguing that what may look like a selfless act is really gratifying to one's egotism and a disguised grab for power. This is one example of Nietzsche's anticipation of the concept of compromise formations. Nietzsche termed himself a psychologist, turning in disgust away from the philosophizing that he saw as palliative and irrelevant. Provocatively proclaiming the death of God, he sought to emphasize the individual's direct relationship to the world and particularly his responsibility in determining an ethical code of behavior for himself.

The subjective criteria for doing so was Nietzsche's (1887) concept of the "eternal return of the same." Here Nietzsche advises that one's actions ought to be predicated on being able to desire that every moment of one's life be repeated an infinite number of times.

"Philosophizing with a hammer," Nietzsche wished to smash the assumption that we can have access to the Universal, a notion that is basic to the "transcendental analytic," Kant's legacy that had so influenced enlightenment thought. Nietzsche objected to the dominance of the Platonic ideal in the philosophy of his time. Briefly, the Platonic ideal argues that ideal forms exist for everything conceivable. These are available to us only through thought, and we come to know anything through a comparison of what we observe around us with these nonphysical, ideal forms. This kind of ideality is expressed in Kant's transcendental analysis, as he relies on an ideal form and what Nietzsche took to be a fantasy: the Universal. Among Nietzsche's objections was that such a pervasive concept of our relationship to the world works to prevent us from becoming more fully aware of ourselves as agents in the here and now.

Many regard this destruction of the Kantian transcendental and the undermining of Platonic ideality as providing a philosophical basis for the disastrous political events that destroyed millions of lives. Others argue that Nietzsche was appalled at the nationalism promoted in his name by his sister and that he would have repudiated Nazism (e.g., Kaufmann, 1968). But the shift from a locus of judgment that is exterior to one that is interior and the assumption of the responsibilities that follow from this move remains, to some degree, an aim of psychoanalytic work and value in psychoanalytic thought. This relationship between an inner and outer locus of ethical judgment can also be thought of as a description of the dominant narrative strand in the philosophy of ethics.

Although it has been persuasively argued that psychoanalysis presents a convincing naturalistic description of ethical development (Scheffler, 1992), leaving behind both Kantian and Nietzschean ideas, two notable problems remain. One is the tendency for the emphasis on ethics in psychoanalytic literature to remain consistently focused on the development of a patient's ethical sense, leaving the analyst's explicit ethical choices and dilemmas out of the picture. The second is that Kantian and Nietzschean ideas do make appearances in psychoanalytic literature, both explicitly and implicitly. I propose that observing the oscillating relationship between the Kantian and Nietzschean ethical points of view can be a useful way of looking at the construction of the ethical stance of the psychoanalyst as expressed in our theory and practice.

Both the Kantian transcendental and the subjective, experiential descriptions of an ethical grounding are implicit in certain examples of classical literature, but the emphasis consistently is placed on the outcomes for the patient. It is as if certain aspects of the psychoanalytic situation, notably those associated with the vulnerability of the analyst, are suppressed. This suppression has assumed the form of certain theories of technique, particularly with regard to the analytic frame. What I am arguing here is that this suppression has the potential to lead to situations in which the analyst may be in an ethically uncomfortable position in both a Kantian and a Nietzschean schema.

ETHICS IN PSYCHOANALYSIS AND THE CONSTRUCTION OF THE ANALYST

In certain examples of the classical psychoanalytic literature, psychoanalysis is regarded as "a secular 'cure of souls'" in which "processes of an ethical and religious kind work together and are indispensable" (Levy-Suhl, 1947, p. 110). And, I would add, the medium of psychoanalytic wisdom, the analyst, having been analyzed, is thus constructed and comes to be known as the embodiment of ethical maturity. For Levy-Suhl, psychoanalytic treatment makes up "for omissions of an ethical and religious kind" (p. 116). He compares the ethical ramifications of the work of Freud and Kant: "Just as Kant arrived at this principle of the autonomy of morality when at the height of his investigations . . . so in the same way Freud came, after decades of successful application of the pleasure principle . . . to the recognition that there existed mental modes of behavior beyond the pleasure principle" (p. 112).

By 1952 the British analyst, Money-Kyrle, expressing the empiricist ideals of the period, argued that psychoanalysis could effect a "transfer of an ethical problem from philosophy to science" (p. 225). Proposing a taxonomy of moral types, he sought to demonstrate that through the use of psychoanalysis as a method of research, "we have discovered that there is a causal link between the possession of a certain kind of conscience and the possession of a certain kind of wisdom" (p. 232). This kind of wisdom he terms humanist. Money-Kyrle's humanism is strongly inflected by a Nietzschean point of view: "The humanists are influenced more by positive loyalties than by restrictive codes" (p. 233). This note of Nietzschean individualism is a distinctive strain in so explicitly empiricist an ideal. We can understand how strongly psychoanalysts writing in the aftermath of World War II may have wished to be able to predict their role in preventing the recurrence of an event that seemed so brutally contemptuous of individual ethics and efficacy. Striving toward such a confident assertion, Money-Kyrle (1952) goes so far as to argue that "the effect of increasing insight [through psychoanalysis] would be to bring about some convergence in political ideology towards what may still be called, in spite of totalitarian attempts to misappropriate the term, the democratic aim" (p. 234). Kant's Categorical Imperative is once again implicitly invoked, as the democratic aim is seen as a logical outcome of psychoanalytic treatment. And the burden shouldered by psychoanalytic treatment, and thus by psychoanalysts themselves, extends from the ethical behavior of the individual to that of political entities.

Two works published in the same year take up the contrasting Kantian and Nietzschean points of view. Hartmann (1960), writing in a Kantian transcendentalist mode, argues that "psychoanalysis as a psychology of the central problems of personality, is naturally in constant contact with the moral feeling and moral judgement of man" (pp. 9–10). Hartmann sharply distinguishes between the necessity of assuming a technically neutral moral stance and ultimate questions of right and wrong. What is morally right is not an illusion, but neither is its quality available to scientific, including psychoanalytic, description. Hartmann regards it as possible, indeed necessary, for the analyst to refrain from articulating his own philosophical point of view, "camouflaged with analytic terminology," in the treatment (p. 24). Here the theory of therapeutic action of the drive-conflict model, conceived within a Kantian point of view, works to create the version of the analyst who, while remaining anonymous and transparent, furthers the maturation (including the ethical maturation) of the patient.

Writing in the same year, Nielson (1960) points out that the "overwhelming importance of value judgments in therapeutic work and in theory formation . . . often seem to be taken for granted and more or less consciously accepted" (p. 245). He argues for greater attention to the moral values that are inevitably imparted through the treatment. Like Nietzsche, he denies that it is possible or even desirable *not* to express one's moral values. We must embrace our convictions rather than pretend that they can be set aside. However, while Nielson draws attention to the ethical and moral ground upon which psychoanalysis exists, the relationship between psychoanalysis and ethics remains a transparent, apparently unconflicted, one.

Subsequent literature, written to a degree under the influence of the classical tradition, continues to observe how psychoanalytic treatment affects a development of higher order ethics. Erikson, (1964, 1976), Racker (1966), Eckstein (1976), Serota (1976), Wallerstein (1976) and Meissner, (1994), all urge psychoanalysts to embrace that aspect of the therapeutic relationship in which ethical values are enhanced. These analysts' arguments attempt, in varying ways, a conciliation of the Kantian and Nietzschean points of view. This reflects the enduring influence of the classical theory of mind and a theory of therapeutic action on which it is based. Once the infantile conflicts have been resolved in the natural unfolding of the analysis of the transference, patients will be able to function with a greater degree of freedom and creativity. Ethical decisions will not be made according to a primitive system of retaliation or by blindly following rules set by others. Kant's legacy remains manifest in this literature's characterization of psychoanalysis as a science with natural outcomes, where the analyst's contribution must be minimized. Nietzsche's influence hovers nonetheless in the characterization of the psychoanalytic process as defiant of conformity and emphasizing the flowering of the patient's individuality.

But what of the analyst's idealizations and identifications related to an ethical and moral ground? As the facilitator of the patient's ethical development, the analyst functions both as a healer and a teacher. An exploration of the analyst's identification with the Hippocratic Oath, revealing "idealized images . . . demonstrable in the classic model of the analyst," posits "common tendencies to masochistic enactment and intellectual inhibition . . . [that] often go unanalyzed because of their ego-syntonic presence in the cultural and ego ideal of the good physician" (McLaughlin, 1961, p. 106). Describing the "relatedness between the individual dynamisms of the analyst and those implicit to the cultural identity of the healer" (p. 107), McLaughlin's context is a detailed analysis of the ancient Greek myth of Aesculapius, the prototypical healer who was destroyed by Zeus for his hubris. McLaughlin sees in the identity of the ideal analyst a compromise formation that defends against vengeful wishes toward the father, as well as a generalized renunciation of aggressive expression or gratification. Analysts often present an "ego-syntonic role enactment of the good doctor: he is either solicitous or exhausted" (p. 119).

McLaughlin's analysis is written in a traditionally Freudian mode, and so the description of relationships between analyst and patient does not consider the mutual influence pursuant to such idealizations. The analyst's power in relation to patients is implicated in the description of the idealized identity of the healer that the community requires, but the fact of the analyst's dependence on patients for his or her livelihood is neglected. By analyzing the central importance of renunciation in the identity of the analyst, the burden of idealized representations is discussed in such a way as to approve and reinforce these idealizations and to deny the element of the analyst's actual and fantasied dependence on others for the maintenance of that identity. (For a detailed analysis of the medical model that provided an ideal for many psychoanalysts prior to the relational turn, see Stepansky, 1999.)

THEORETICAL INNOVATION, ETHICS, AND IDEALIZATION

Psychoanalytic theories have posited the achievement of higher order ethical relating as a developmental process. Ideas that were initially presented as philosophical concepts became translated into psychological and developmental phenomena. The analyst is positioned as helping the analysand to attain these developmental goals. It has been taken for granted that the analyst's ethical development is already established from his or her own analysis during training. This ideal joins other dynamic idealizations of the analyst. In this process of idealization, the ethical dimension of the analyst's activity is obscured as clinical issues dominate the foreground.

The challenge, then, is to tease out the analyst's ethical position from a theory focused on the psychology and development of the patient. Sometimes this seems an unlikely project where incompatible methods of observation and analysis knock up against each other. For example, Nietzsche's (1887) exhortations for honesty about humanity's basic selfishness, the "will to power" to which even an analyst is vulnerable, seem to evade or ignore values of human relatedness that are observed most obviously in the infant–mother dyad and that are crucial to psychoanalytic thinking. But this understanding neglects Nietzsche's concept of "the eternal return of the same." To *desire* that every moment of one's life be repeated an infinite number of times—without masochism, without guilt, without renunciation—surely implies the kind of mutuality that characterizes developed interpersonal relations.

Taking up Kant's Imperative to regard every individual as an end rather than as a means to an end could be thought of as another description of mutuality: the capacity to relate to others as subjects, not as objects. Psychoanalytic theory offers various examples of this concept as taking place through a developmental process. It is a shift from a narcissistic to an object-oriented mode of relating. Klein (1957) described this as the move from the paranoid/schizoid position to the depressive position. In a self-psychological framework it is seen as developing the capacity to see others as functioning less as selfobjects than as individuals with selfobject needs of their own. But the analyst too must be regarded as an end in himself, and not only as the means through which the patient achieves this condition.

Psychoanalysis has made odd bedfellows of philosophers whose ideas clashed vividly. It is almost as if a combination of Kant's Imperative and Nietzsche's eternal return of the same, in a sort of figure/ground relationship, is implied in this description of highly developed ethical relations, one that allows for an ever greater subtlety with regard to developmental paradigms. Examples of more nuanced developmental narratives are those that detail a more complicated subjectivity for mothers (e.g., Benjamin, 1988; Kraemer, 1996), as well as for infants (e.g., Stern, 1985).

The importance of an ever-refined developmental narrative has exerted profound influences on psychoanalytic technique, with relevant effects on an ethical stance for the analyst. When Mitchell (1988b) described "the developmental tilt" in psychoanalysis, he urged analysts not to see analysands as infants. In the interim, analytic writers have developed theories of multiplicity of subjective experience, making room for developmental narratives along with other stories. But the apprehension, for example, that a disclosure concerning the analyst's private life might be too burdensome, can slide down a "developmental tilt." The analogy here is to the caregiver's role in protecting the infant from too much stimulation prior to the development of the infant's ego functioning. As more sophisticated infant development studies provided a new, more scientific narrative, the directive to avoid self-disclosure lost its justification of maintaining a blank screen. But as the developmental studies provided us with a naturalistic basis for a two-person model of psychic functioning, the technical proscriptions regarding disclosure have been retheorized from a developmental point of view, with the same result. Developmental studies are based on, and in turn confirm, a naturalizing of the parental metaphor for the analyst.

Some of the growing literature of intersubjectivity theory describes a movement away from the developmental tilt, without neglecting developmental concerns altogether (see Teicholz, 1999). At the same time, some of the latent ethical bases are reconsidered as well. The capacity to acknowledge the deep subjectivity of another individual, however this may be observed or operationalized, has risen to the status of the sine qua non of progress in treatment and psychological health.

Our psychoanalytic telos has shifted from the ability to love and work, picking up the capacity to play during psychoanalysis' British efflorescence, to a far more detailed description of relating between the two subjects of the analytic encounter. Examples of this literature are numerous, transcending boundaries of theoretical orientation. Philosophers such as Thomas Nagel (1986) anticipate some of this literature's language of perspectivalism (e.g., Orange, 1995). His description of the capacity to detach from a particular perspective and to transcend one's time and place sounds exactly like what many of the people who come to psychoanalysts to relieve their suffering *cannot* do.

For this reason, it appears that psychoanalysts are inevitably placed in a position where we must conduct ourselves with a degree of relativism with regard to ethics. Particularly at the beginning of a treatment, the partners are *not* equal. However much we "put our cards on the table" (Renik, 1999), however much we behave as if we are equal partners, the power of transference tends to shift power in our direction. And here we must contend with a theory that is necessarily pragmatic: what is it that works, how and why, and who decides? How mindful ought we to be not only of the clinical, but also the ethical constituent of the ground against which we assess what works, and why? To what extent is the analyst's entitlement to a private life in tension with those ethical concerns that are part of the ground on which the treatment relationship unfolds?

Several components of the psychoanalytic situation—accumulated clinical knowledge, the analyst's own idealizations of his or her identity, and the metaphor of the parent—contribute to an implicit ethical role for the analyst. The literature and the codes of ethics that attempt to address certain themes paradoxically reinscribe an idealization of the analyst, even as they are designed to protect against the effects of that idealization. This reinscription depends on a process of hiding or dissociating the inevitable vulnerabilities of the analyst, covering this process in theories and technical recommendations based on those theories.

The situation in which I found myself when I met with Jack prompted me to ask a question about the frame and the ethical condition of the analyst from a different angle. Do certain recommendations with regard to the analytic frame have the potential to place the analyst in an ethically untenable position in relation both to the patient and to himself? The implications of the classic literature, that the analyst is the medium and example of the advanced ethical development that is the outcome of analytic treatment, place the analyst in the position of godlike invulnerability. Important literature has accumulated recently concerning examples of acting out, such as engaging in sexual relationships with patients (e.g., Gabbard and Lester, 1995; Davies, 2000; Pizer, 2000). But the underlying condition of ethical dissonance with regard to the inherent vulnerability of the analyst's position remains unaddressed. Particularly in a situation of the analyst's illness and death is this gap apparent.

In Jack's case, did his former analyst's strict maintenance of the rule concerning nondisclosure of personal information lead to a situation in which *both* Jack and his analyst were treated in ways that, arguably, are unethical? From a Kantian point of view, I suggest that by not informing Jack about the truth of her situation, the analyst not only failed to treat Jack as an end in himself, but, also, by inadvertently treating another person in this way, she failed to treat herself as an end in herself. The technical advice to refrain from making personal disclosures left her unavoidably treating a patient badly, a course of events I feel certain that no analyst would desire. And, I contend, no person would wish this on herself.

From the Nietzschean point of view in which every moment of life ought to be lived in such a way that we'd desire it to be repeated an infinite number of times, the subjective is emphasized. The only criterion is the person's considered conviction. I do not wish to put myself in the untenable position of suggesting how another person ought to make such a decision, let alone to repeat such a moment an infinite number of times. I do know, having withheld the truth about a medical condition from a patient, that it is a moment I do not wish to repeat infinitely.

What I believe I sought to prevent, in making a disclosure to Jack at the very outset of our work together, was a repetition of the dissociation of the analyst's vulnerability as well as the prospective patient's. This dissociation, this setting aside, is disguised by the legacy of technical advice and classic theory, as well as by contemporary intersubjective theory that emphasizes the power of the analyst's authoritative position. This emphasis is one manifestation of the naturalizing of the analyst's role through the parental metaphor. I do not argue for trying to counter the effects of this metaphor. Such a move would be impossible, let alone clinically counterproductive. What I do believe is that the uses the prospective patient will make of the analyst's subjectivity, once the treatment has begun, will not be inhibited by such a disclosure. More positively, the grounding of a treatment begun in an ethically intersubjective manner will contribute to the effective engagement of the treatment, in that the analyst will be unencumbered by the knowledge of keeping hidden information that is potentially relevant to the treatment relationship.

As Greenberg (1995) points out, every disclosure is predicated on a tacit decision *not* to disclose something else. We have no choice but to participate in the setting aside of one thing when we do, or decide not to do, another. We will never know what opportunities for gaining clinical traction with Jack were lost once I disclosed my HIV status. What the two of us were able to learn about was the tendency we had together to set aside how desire and death underlay what seemed at first to be the most casual moments of our interactions. It is a trade that I now feel is worth making.

CHAPTER 5

OTHER ANALYSTS' EXPERIENCES

IN THE SPRING OF 1997, I offered a workshop called "The HIV-Positive Therapist" at the annual conference of the Institute for Human Identity in New York City. I was aware that listing my name in the announcement of the conference's schedule was itself a disclosure, and that the possibility that patients of mine would see this announcement made this action, in the estimation of some, an example of acting out. This conference has traditionally offered experiential and supportive workshops in addition to didactic and theoretical ones, and it seemed an important opportunity to begin to counteract what I experienced as the invisibility of the HIV-positive analyst in the professional community.

At that first workshop, among the small group who attended were some therapists who had been analytically trained. That afternoon we explored several questions, including whether and how to disclose our HIV status to patients, the potential effects of disclosure on our work with patients who are also HIV positive, and the potential effects on work with those who aren't. Perhaps most important, though, was a feeling that we could describe those specific aspects of our experiences that pertain to HIV both within and beyond the context of our clinical work. Some of the participants at that workshop said that it was important to them not to reveal their serostatus in their work settings, which included not telling their supervisors, for fear that this information could have a negative impact on their positions. Their relief at being able to discuss this and other fears was palpable.

Because not all of those who attended the workshop had been analytically trained, there were widely divergent attitudes and degrees of experience concerning matters having to do with the transference–countertransference matrix, analytic anonymity, and disclosure. The discussion of clinical aspects of our common dilemma foundered, somewhat, on a lack of common experience with, and knowledge of, a body of literature and theory, and the attempt to come to terms with the technical recommendations that make up part of the psychoanalytic discourse. For example, one participant wondered why we would have any hesitations about making the disclosure of HIV status. He was used to working in a counseling model that does not emphasize transference–countertransference considerations. (Interestingly, after asserting that he routinely informed all of the people he worked with of his serostatus, he told us that he'd suddenly realized that this was not accurate, and that there was an unconscious process of selection guiding his disclosures. He stated that it was useful to him to come to this understanding.) Though our exchange on the experience of working in a mental health setting as an HIV-positive person was generally helpful and relieving, the misunderstandings resulting from our divergent backgrounds and theoretical orientations pointed up how widely varied our needs and concerns were. Also, it was apparent that our particular needs and concerns were determined, to a certain extent, by and through the different sorts of training we'd had and the range of our theoretical orientations.

For these reasons, when it came time to plan a focused, sustained exploration of the experience of the HIV-positive analyst, I decided that it was important to specify that prospective respondents be analytically trained so that I could rely on a baseline of familiarity with some analytic literature on disclosure, transference and countertransference, and standard technique.

THE SEARCH FOR SUBJECTS

Two years after that first workshop, I began the search for HIV-positive analysts, a group whom I could interview for this inquiry into the influence and experience of the analyst's seropositivity on psychoanalytic therapy. I wrote letters to 50 persons, including members of a professional society in New York City called GALA (Gay and Lesbian Analysts). The membership of this society comes from a wide range of theoretical orientations and training institutes. In my letter, I described the research I wished to do and how I planned to do it. I asked the recipients of my letters if they knew any HIV-positive analysts and if they felt comfortable telling them about my planned study. I received no response.

I directed another letter, along with a brief description of the proposed study to post on bulletin boards, to the chairpersons of professional societies of 30 analytic institutes located in New York, Boston, Philadelphia, Chicago, San Francisco, and Los Angeles. I received no response. Later attempts to follow up via telephone yielded no better results. (The letters and a flyer I sent to psychoanalytic institutes are included as Appendices A–C.)

Several months after these mailings, I was at a meeting of GALA and was approached by an analyst who has written on HIV and psychoanalysis. He is affiliated with an institute in New York City, although he is not the chairperson of the professional society there. My letter had been routed to him, presumably because of his well-known interest in, and expertise with, HIV-related issues. He told me that he was not sure why, exactly, my letter had reached his mailbox, and was not sure what to do with it. I said only that I'd be grateful, were he comfortable with the idea, if he would alert any HIV-positive analysts he knew to my project. Over a year after my first inquiries, I had received no responses to any of these communications searching for interview subjects.

Silence is often as eloquent as speech, from a psychoanalytic perspective. But in the psychoanalytic situation, there is a silent other who eventually confirms or denies hypotheses as to the reasons for a silence. In this situation, I can only report my speculations as to why I received no response to my attempts to make contact with other HIV-positive analysts.

First, and most obvious, it is clear that no one wants to talk about this subject. Why would this be so? Perhaps it is not a very interesting problem any more. Now that we have a number of medications that effectively suppress viral activity for many who take them, it is possible that HIV is no longer a pressing issue for the seropositive analyst. For such persons, HIV is a manageable, chronic condition that makes itself known only when it is time to wolf down a handful of pills or to have blood drawn for quarterly tests. It may be fair to say that it has become the unnoticed background, a nearly invisible part of daily life. However upsetting it may have been to learn of one's seropositive status, as long as one is asymptomatic and the medications are doing what they ought, HIV is nearly not there.

If this is a strong explanation, then we may assume that the meanings associated with HIV infection are also worked through and seem not to be of interest to explore in the context of a research project. Sexuality, transgression, and how these have become linked with death are themes that I have noted exerting significant influence within myself; these are elaborated in the fiction and nonfiction AIDS narratives. (Good examples are the novels and memoirs of Paul Monette, 1988; Edmund White, 1994; David Feinberg, 1995; and Mark Doty, 1996.) I know that for myself, and for those patients I work with now who are positive and stable on the medication cocktail, those themes continue to exert their emotive power in our psychic lives. I am extremely skeptical that these issues are not of interest to psychoanalysts, and at the same time I can understand that it is extremely difficult to imagine exploring them as they manifest in one's own psyche.

No, I don't believe that no one responded to my request because there is nothing to talk about. I believe that no one responded to my request because there is too much to talk about, and the idea of talking to a stranger, fellow psychoanalyst or not, is not a congenial one.

Traditionally, psychoanalysts train their concentration on the psychic lives of others. It was only in the second part of the 20th century that, gradually, the analyst's own emotional life became the object of study, as a source of information of the patient's unconscious life. In the late 1990s, the analyst's private experience became interesting to other analysts, and it was possible to explore how pregnancy, illness, childlessness, disability, age, and other conditions exerted an influence on the clinical lives of analyst and patient (e.g., Gerson, 1996). Perhaps the reticence that makes the analytic job a strain sometimes also makes the idea of talking about a condition like HIV seropositivity seem too great a risk.

What do we risk? I believe that there is a quality of monkish rectitude, a chastity, an innocence, conferred on the analytic role. (In a letter to his friend Fleiss, Freud suggests that he felt relief that, in his mid-forties, his conjugal duties were over. See Freud, 1985, p. 276). Whether we wish it, know it consciously, or not, so we, too, may be construed by our patients, and perhaps there is a part of ourselves that likes this aspect of our role.

In some ways what we do and how we do it contributes to this construction. One element of technique is never to take it for granted that we know what a patient refers to without as many details as it is possible for the patient to give us. In obtaining these details, we often must inquire in such a way as to communicate that we do not know about the experience in question, as if we had not performed a particular sexual act, gone to a certain place, imbibed a particular substance. In such an inquiry, analysts may maintain a neutral, relatively anonymous stance. We indicate neither that we know what it is like to take Ecstasy, to hang out at a singles or back-room bar, or to engage in group sex, nor that we do not know what it is like. We are interested only in what it is like for the patient.

Implicit and explicit in much of the psychoanalytic literature is the assessment that behaviors associated with these places and activities are immature, and that, in the unlikely event that someone who is now an analyst once behaved in such a way, our analyses, if sufficient, would have resolved the character problems that led to our participation in such pastimes. Further, training analyses perform a function that purports to guarantee that our own experiences are not of interest and ought not become part of the analytic process. It is easy to imagine that analysts are thought to be sanitized, hygienic, and certainly never the bearers of a potentially deadly virus that is transmitted through bodily fluids and acts of interpenetration. The effect of certain fantasies concerning our training analyses, whether they are our own or our patients', is that the analyst is often construed as remaining innocent of those aspects of human life that are categorized as transgressive. Conversely, the analyst is representative of those aspects of human life that are categorized as normative and authoritative. After all, in many, if not in all treatments, at least some of the time, we stand in for parents, often as idealized ones.

If this air of chaste rectitude is a part of the analytic frame, an aspect of the treatment relationship that enables clinical progress by focusing attention on the patient's difficulties, the idealizing quality that the analytic frame can impart to the treatment relationship exerts an influence on the analyst as well. In the extreme, it can become the source of a rather obsessive, if not paranoid, concern. For example, in a conversation about the potential for unconsciously making disclosures by leaving items in plain sight in the office, a colleague described being careful not to leave certain books where a patient might see them. I had told him of leaving a book about AIDS on the footstool by my chair, which a patient noticed and inquired about. My colleague asked me whether I might unconsciously have wished to tell this patient that I am HIV positive.

Though it may be true that I unconsciously wished to make this disclosure, the perception of the need to hide an object such as a book discloses something, too. Some time ago, in those years when I did make sure that I left no books where patients would assume that I'd been reading them, I noticed that I felt distinctly like a criminal or a naughty child, covering up incriminating traces of some kind. Rather than controlling for an inadvertent disclosure, I felt controlled by my need to remain unsullied in the patient's estimation.

Here is an example of how an unremarkable aspect of standard technique, maintaining the relative anonymity customary to the analyst's role, took on a paranoid quality. I found it necessary to keep my *reading material* a secret from patients. What does this express about our attitudes toward ourselves? About our patients? Eventually I wished no longer to feel, or to communicate indirectly, that something such as a book I might be reading is somehow off limits, and beyond our capacity to analyze together. Generally, it has been my experience that such matters are available to analysis, including my acknowledgment that a topic such as AIDS is of interest to me for a variety of reasons, as it may be to many people. Any fantasies generated by a book a patient notices, like any other item in my office that sparks a comment, have been useful, opening into elaborations of the analysis of our relationship.

If, as Blechner (1997a) and Schaffner (cited in Blechner, 1997a) report, there was at one time a stigma in the analytic community attached to *treating* HIV-positive patients, it does not seem unlikely that there remains a stigma attached to *being* an HIV-positive person in this community. It is commonly accepted that the stigma associated with HIV infection, for a gay man, has to do with promiscuous sex. The openly HIV-positive psychoanalyst (and even possibly the HIV-positive psychoanalyst willing to talk about this condition for an anonymous research study) confronts the image of the austere, chaste, ideal analyst, and how he does not live up to this ideal.

This ideal is composed of a matched, gendered, parental couple. The fully analyzed father is the one who has been able to develop ways to express important needs in as conscious a manner as possible. The one who has, with Freud, replaced *id* with *ego*. When preoedipal experience was opened up and the experiences of infancy became of greater importance, the psychoanalytic role was modified and naturalized by the maternal metaphor. This metaphor expresses a certain investment in monogamy. That original dyad persists in spite of the shifting identities of actual lovers over time. In classical theory, psychic maturity is measured by the extent to which new love objects are no longer merely replacements or substitutes for the original love object. Just how truly new that new love object may be is based on the quality of the relationship: whether the individual has truly attained genitality, having renounced the gratification associated with the infant–mother pair (e.g., Blos, 1967). This emphasis on renunciation of the mother heightens her presence even in the contemporary, revised psychoanalytic narrative. The two members of the analytic dyad, one that often is described as replicating the mother–infant pair, remain true to one another. Implicit in this structure is the notion that it is this monogamous pair that expresses what is most *natural and good* in human relationships.

Here is one source of the psychoanalytic critique of relationships that do not so pattern themselves. Serial monogamy, for example, is suspect because the relationships do not last. It is assumed, often, that the partners cannot tolerate the frustrations inherent in any human relationship, and thus that they are immature, prone to replacing love objects that have proven to be disappointing. The valuing of monogamy in psychoanalytic theory is so pervasive that to offer other explanations for the supremacy of long-term, monogamous relationships in our culture, and, more to the point, *supporting* alternative arrangements that patients (or analysts) might devise, is highly suspect.

Because of the prolonged immaturity of the human infant and the steadfast caretaking that mother and child require, the nuclear family has come to represent not only the natural, but the optimally healthy. But through history there have been other familial structures providing an environment that enabled human infants to develop to adulthood. To suggest an alternative explanation for our current cultural preference for a particular family unit renders an analyst vulnerable to accusations of superficially undervaluing what has come to be regarded as bedrock in our theory. For example, an economic explanation might argue that smaller nuclear family units are more dependent on the market economy of consumer capitalism and so more controllable, leading to the social preference and enforcement of what we recognize as a conventional family structure. If we were to include a materialist understanding of the construction of the family in the development of our psychic lives, would that undermine our sense of the primacy of psychoanalytic theory? Or is there a way to take into account explanations for certain motivations and idealizations in addition to the powerful maternal metaphor and the ensuing emphasis on monogamy?

The HIV-positive psychoanalyst willing to talk about his HIV seropositivity risks the internal and external tensions of defying an idealized image rooted in the narrative of the "natural," and thus

"healthy," family unit as it is known in our culture. One of the lega-
cies of AIDS has been the domestication of the homosexual. As a
demographic group, we demonstrated our maturity in the years of
unrelenting horror by organizing, mourning, and, most importantly,
learning how not to spread HIV by altering our sexual behavior.
For many, this change in sexual behavior has meant an end to multiple, casual sexual contacts. Other, rather notorious, activists insist
that it is not reducing the number of sexual partners that makes for
greater safety, but the specific activities that sex partners engage in
that must be safer. However, those whose voices make up the side
of the argument that does not advocate striving for monogamy and
commitment tend to be regarded at best as immature, and at worst,
as actively spreading disease. It is nearly unacceptable, even within
parts of the gay community, to question a trend toward the "normal," by which we mean the heterosexual nuclear family, because
this would be understood as saying that we hadn't learned anything
from the last 20 years of life with AIDS. (For an analysis of this
argument and a detailed presentation of the view against striving
for the "normal," see Warner, 1999.)

The analyst who contracted HIV sexually must contend with
the effects of an idealization of the role of analyst that may be one
of his own psychic representations and perhaps was a constitutive
identification that led to the choice of doing analysis as a career.
This is an additional burden to the already highly charged feelings
about becoming HIV positive in the first place. However the person comes to terms with the fact of being positive in a private sphere
of experience, being a psychoanalyst presents an additional inner
negotiation of meanings. In addition to sharing personal medical
information with a stranger, the analyst willing to talk about HIV-
positive serostatus is once again vulnerable, not only to his own
feelings about having seroconverted, but also possibly to questions
about how this clashes with a psychic representation of himself as
psychoanalyst. Those who present themselves as interested in relieving the suffering of others may have a range of reasons to experience themselves as free of suffering of their own (see Schwartz and
Silver, 1990, for descriptions of the fantasy of the analyst's training analysis as inoculation).

HIV-Positive Psychoanalysts Willing to Talk

At professional gatherings, I was fortunate enough to meet three psychoanalysts who let me know that they are HIV positive. All three are gay men who have, over their years in practice, treated a significant number of homosexual males who were coping with the spectrum of HIV/ AIDS. All agreed immediately to my request for tape-recorded interviews. I am grateful for their willingness to participate and for their brave candor in describing intimate feelings and experiences from their personal and clinical lives.

The material related to me in those interviews was unusual not only because it is about seropositive psychoanalysts, but also because of the intimate quality of much of my coresearchers' reflections. The quality of mutual inquiry that dominates the process of a heuristic study leads me to use the rather clumsy term coresearcher. It is common in the psychoanalytic literature to read of patients' sexual, envious, and aggressive wishes and fantasies. It is exceptional to read of these feelings as they occur on the other side of the couch. Although it has been acknowledged from the early days of the practice that psychoanalysts will feel such feelings, it is very rare for them to be fleshed out in detail. As Pizer (2000) has put it, psychoanalysts are emerging from behind the curtain, to be revealed in all their flawed humanity. The added condition of HIV seropositivity prompted an expression of wishes and feelings from these psychoanalysts that presented a heightened struggle to honestly face such feelings as lust, envy, and aggression, and to go on finding ways to work effectively with their own patients.

Whether it might be useful to generalize about HIV-positive psychoanalysts from the experiences that my colleagues described in these interviews is a claim I do not wish to make. I offer this analysis knowing that I will reveal more about how my impressions are formed than about what being HIV positive means to them. My imagination was stimulated by the intimate reflections that my co-researchers shared with me concerning the relationship they described between their serostatus and their work at a given moment in time. Two of them described thoughts and fantasies very similar to my own on the subject of the meanings of being HIV positive: stigma and transgressive sexuality. All four of us have in common a sense of shifting attitudes about being positive in the years since we tested. For all that we have in common, though, what interests me most are the differences in our experiences of seropositivity and clinical work. Though there may be areas of such commonality as to constitute a generalizable experience of the HIV-positive analyst, it may be that more insight is available through the accumulation of differences, rather than a distillation of sameness. It was striking to me that each of these subjects remarked, in one way or another, that they had not had an opportunity to discuss in detail certain questions with other seropositive colleagues. So it is to be hoped that what is presented here is the beginning of a process for all of us, rather than a description of a stable, worked-through condition or identity.

The interviews took place several months apart. One was held in my office, another in the office of the subject, and the third in the home of the subject. Each interview lasted 90 minutes. The interviews were structured only to the extent that I prepared eight questions to provide a way of beginning. In each interview we freely departed from this list as the subjects' associations ranged where they would. The questions began with such closed-ended questions as: "How long have you known you were HIV positive?" The other questions I was prepared to ask each subject were purposefully devised to encourage reflection and an accumulation of associations. These questions were:

- Can you describe your thoughts about being positive? Have your thoughts about being positive changed over time?
- Has your being positive explicitly figured into your work with patients, and how?
- Do you think being positive has figured implicitly in your work with patients, and how?
- Has being positive changed your work with patients in some way?
- Do you think being positive is something that increases and decreases in your experience doing clinical work?

– Is it possible to describe when or how your being positive increases or decreases in importance or awareness doing clinical work?"

I participated freely as well, offering my own responses and experiences. My intention was to allow as much imaginative free play around the question of our HIV status and its implications in our work as possible.

Much of the more immediate affective life that was revealed in each subject's remarks was not focused on HIV specifically but was expressed in other images or memories that were articulated in the interviews. The psychoanalytic concept of displacement, whereby feelings associated with one situation are shifted to another, may be relevant here. Interpretations of the material that is discussed along these lines are necessarily filtered through my subjective experience of these conversations. In the spirit of psychoanalytic interpretations, these hypotheses are offered only as suggestions to promote further thought, not as definitive explanations. Although we shared a condition, an identity of sorts, it became clear that the ways we've each interpreted the meanings of this condition, this identity, are widely divergent. The content of the experiences associated with our HIV seropositivity and working as psychoanalysts is elaborated so variously as to challenge any notion that there is a persistent, lasting, essence to the experience of HIV seropositivity.

ON THE PROBLEM OF PRESENTING COLLEAGUES' MATERIAL, AND METHODS OF ANALYSIS

An earlier version of this chapter included an anonymous demographic description of the group of interview subjects and direct quotations from portions of the interviews. The material was rich and intimate, and I was enthusiastic about a presenting my colleagues' candid explorations. Because of the extremely small size of the sample, the research model often used in psychoanalysis—the single case study—was most appropriate (Edelson, 1984). Rarely have psychoanalysts themselves openly been subjects of qualitative research. It has seemed to me that traditionally, psychoanalysts have derived some of their power from their opacity, remaining unknown. A presentation of some of what my coresearchers discussed with me was a way to counter that tradition. I hoped to contribute to a greater openness about psychoanalysis through an intimate description of the analyst's experience.

However, the style of that initial presentation and the method of analysis placed my colleagues and me in an untenable situation. First, the question of guaranteeing the anonymity of my coresearchers was felt to be extremely problematic. Because of the size of the group and the relatively small number of psychoanalysts in the general population, there seemed to be no effective way to disguise the identities of my coresearchers. Even the men's particular manners of speech (their verbal idioms) could not be sufficiently disguised. It was felt that personalities could be discernable through the direct quotations, inviting readers into the sort of peek-a-boo game that makes the roman à clef so compelling. This atmosphere of risk prevented including extensive quotation. Disguises of various sorts were rejected as well, because none felt sufficiently protective and these tended to seem false, particularly in an enterprise grounded in being candid.

That we all risk something emphasizes one of the most pervasive themes saturating any discussion of HIV, even 20 years into the history of the syndrome. Owing to this sense of risk, the verbatim presentation of another's construction of meanings of HIV seropositivity, articulated in highly idiosyncratic ways, will remain beyond the scope of this project. This is the property of each person, and it must remain up to each participant whether and how to present his own story.

Also uncomfortable was my position as the interpreter of my colleagues' material, a necessary role in the single case-study model. Here I confronted the problem of the relationship between the text—the ongoing construction of personal meaning of HIV seropositivity and doing psychoanalysis—and the context—the edifice of psychoanalytic culture. This is a relationship without clearly demarcated boundaries, as I hope the preceding chapters have shown. Working within the model of the single-case study, I seemed unavoidably to slide into the role of arbiter of meaning, despite my best efforts to present my colleagues' material in as direct a manner as possible. The boundary between doing research and presumptuously becoming analyst to my coresearchers kept melting away as I attempted to analyze the data.

Further, it is arguable that other psychoanalysts' experiences of HIV seropositivity in the context of doing psychoanalysis are too multiply determined to depict in a meaningful way. To say anything with conviction about the meanings of HIV seropositivity depends on a presumption about my colleagues' experiences that I could not comfortably maintain. Like the virus's action within the body, whatever meanings we might convincingly argue do pertain to HIV in particular disperse and adhere to a great many other foci of conscious and unconscious conflict and self-definition.

More to the point, if it were possible to present verbatim transcripts, would this indeed present others' experiences? The conversations I had with my coresearchers are all partially determined by various factors. I composed a list of questions, imposing certain themes that are pressing for me, perhaps less so for others. Unless the entire transcripts were to be presented, allowing readers to interpret the interviews for themselves, I would be making choices of what to include and what to suppress, reflecting far more about what HIV seropositivity means to me than what it means to the participants. The most convincing position available to the researcher in this situation is that the interpretation of the data will reveal something about the researcher, rather his subjects. Proclaiming the death of the author, Barthes (1970) argued that texts are written in the minds of the reader each time they are read. Meaning can no longer be thought of as fixed even though the words conveying it are printed on a page. Meaning circulates endlessly, guided by signs provided by the author, interpreted by the reader. Similarly, the waning of our confidence in an omniscient, objective researcher emphasizes the importance of including the researcher as an object of study. (Indeed, Freud's [1900] prescient *The Interpretation of Dreams*, in which he presented his own dreams, predicted this postmodern turn in psychological research.) If the data to be presented can be approached like a text to be interpreted, these interpretations must themselves be approached as a text that reveals the interpreter. Rather than speculate on an anatomy of meaning, then, I present an interpretation of the construction of the forms that the shifting, mutating meanings took in the moments of the interviews.

A Composite Portrait

Following one heuristic research method devised by Moustakas (1990, pp. 51–52), I first present a depiction of what we as a group of coresearchers shared. This is the outcome of Moustakas's first step, an imaginative immersion into the material gathered throughout the research process. The heuristic researcher seeks a deep empathic connection to the data. The desired culmination of this period of immersion is an expression of themes and experiences that are generalizable to us as a group.

We all participate in an ongoing struggle with the stigma associated with HIV. Some of us experience this as linked to, and as recapitulating, the conflicting attitudes of psychoanalysis toward homosexuality, and our culture's attitude toward homosexuality as well. Each of the interviews includes an analogy along the lines of, "This makes me think of the problems gay analysts who came before us had in dealing with their sexuality." This struggle is particularly acute as we consider the question of disclosing our serostatus, either to our patients or to our colleagues. Whether we feel that this might help or hinder our work with patients turns out to have much more to do with where on the spectrum of theoretical orientation we situate ourselves than with divergent feelings about the virus. If in our work we tend to include disclosures about ourselves or our feelings, we tend to be more inclined to do so about our serostatus as well.

Disclosure of a spoiled identity (Goffman, 1963) such as HIV positivity, undoubtedly complicates the relational field of the clinical situation, and also our daily lives beyond our offices. Even within the gay community, there may be many ways that HIV seropositivity is denoted, announced, or hidden. One paradoxical effect of HIV seropositivity occurs when this particular stigma functions to create an in-group of HIV-positive people perceived as deserving of more attention. The burden of the HIV-negative often is their sense that their feelings of resentment for the care and attention that positives receive are unacceptable (Odets, 1995). For psychoanalysts who are gay and HIV positive, the situation is quite different in that receiving special care is not consonant with the role. Instead, there is simply the residual condition of bearing a double stigma. Some of these themes were apparent as we discussed the question of disclosing our HIV status in various contexts. For example, the potential ramifications of becoming known as HIV positive among our professional colleagues included a worry that our referral sources would be less inclined to send us patients.

Two of us feel that HIV has become an aspect of our identities, that it becomes a part of one's personality. Two of us feel entirely the opposite, that HIV seropositivity does not itself constitute a new identity. This point of view is held by one analyst who discloses, and by another who does not. This suggests that the experience of HIV as an identity does not determine technical approaches and is not determined by a single theoretical point of view, but rather emanates from the realm of the idiomatic, the intuited. In one case, HIV has been the occasion for a recapitulation of attitudes toward illness that the analyst's family traditionally expressed, that illness is to be ignored at all costs. In this regard, for this person HIV is conspicuous through its absence in his felt identity.

In our clinical work, two of us tend to bracket our HIV seropositivity as much as possible, setting it aside to make sure the needs of the analyst do not supercede those of the patient. Two of us do not make this effort. More accurately, we do not believe that bracketing this experience will serve to ensure our focus on our patients. Rather, by including our feelings with regard to our HIV seropositivity freely, we believe that we are serving the same end. This does not imply that we express these feelings to patients, only that we do not seek to set our experience of being HIV positive to one side when we are with patients. These attitudes toward our HIV seropositivity in our work relate to our theories about the role and use of the countertransference, more than to a meaning specific to HIV. But, curiously, one analyst who brackets his HIV experience in his work includes a measure of disclosure of his feelings and experience to his patients. It is pointedly HIV that has a special, bracketed status. The other analyst who brackets HIV in his work tends not to make countertransference or personal disclosures generally. Interestingly, in this small sample, there is no consistent theoretical allegiance that would predict attitudes about whether and how to include HIV seropositivity in our clinical work.

The most pervasive theme in the interviews about our work is how to continue to find ways to be effective with our patients. For all three of my colleagues, their steadfast commitment to finding ways of working effectively, with and because of being HIV positive, is expressed again and again. However intimations of mortality are elaborated for each of these individuals, the importance of being good analysts remains an organizing point of reference; at times it seems to be the one unchanging characteristic known about themselves through perplexing shifts in their health and emotional lives. HIV seropositivity has complicated this task in some ways, but the meanings we construct about our roles as psychoanalysts are far more determinant of our experience than our experience of being HIV positive.

DIFFERENCES AND FORMAL EXPRESSION

As I considered how to approach the problem of presenting the material that expressed the rich variety of how we make meaning out of our common experience, it immediately became clear that my coresearchers's experiences were stories. It is true that these stories—about what they felt when they became aware of their HIV status and what has happened to them since, in their lives and in their clinical work—emerge in a dialogue and in response to my questions, but they are stories nonetheless. Each colleague tells his story in a distinctive idiom, and each story resembles a particular narrative form. The problem confronting this research project, where the participant's need to avoid the presentation of details requires the interposition of a degree of abstraction, necessitates a shift of emphasis from personal detail to that which is symbolically expressed through form. In historical writing about actual human events, Hayden White (1990) has argued that content is expressed by form. If it is fair to think of what my colleagues are sharing with me as stories, as three distinctive narrative histories, one answer to the problem of analysis of this sensitive material is to apply a method pertaining to narrative history.

This method involves presenting the linguisitic data sufficient to differentiating the narratives according to their formal attributes. Units of data smaller than sentences are presented to avoid the risks of extensive direct quotation. These smaller units are often sufficient to convincingly indicate formal attributes. Larger units of data will be presented in a summary, where their inclusion is required to establish the formal characteristics of the narrative. The linguistic data are presented without any accompanying demographic description, once again in the interest of insuring the anonymity of my coresearchers.

This method relies on a theory of historiography set forth by Ricoeur and developed by White. Ricoeur (1984) examines how meaning is produced by sentences where the narrative form carries meaning, rather than looking to metaphor. He posits that meanings of stories are given in their "emplotment," by which events are "configured" or "grasped together" so as to represent symbolically what cannot be put into language (pp. 41–54). White (1990) argues that, because human beings are meaning-making creatures, our narrative discourse will inevitably assume formal attributes. White also finds support for this point of view in a Lacanian model of the registers of psychic experience. In this model, the Real is a register that remains forever beyond our unmediated contact, and we are left with the imaginary and the symbolic as registers of our experience in which we function (see also Bowie, 1991, pp. 99–100). In the imaginary and symbolic registers, the only means we have of encountering our experience is through the construction of a narration of some kind. In that narrative structure we find a meaning that, for thinkers sharing the point of view of Lacan, must be attributed not to the real, referring to the other-than-cultural, but to human culture. Thinking about the construction of personal narratives is a feature of our lives and a way of working with patients that is familiar to psychoanalysts, whether we work in a Lacanian mode or not. It is part of our daily work to point out to a patient the qualities of the stories they tell us about themselves, and that we are enacting together. In psychoanalysis, the specific details may be emphasized, rather than formal structural qualities, or we may look to one to illuminate the other as we work to understand the meanings of these stories.

The analysis of narrative form belongs to the study of literary genres and how genre produces meaning effects, an aspect of the mimetic function of narrative. Ricoeur (1984) turns to Aristotle's *Poetics*, to ground a definition of *mimesis*. Mimesis, imitating or representing action, organizes events through emplotment. Action has priority, the doing. Ricoeur's reading of Aristotle conceives of mimesis in three parts: it refers to a familiar, "pre-understanding we have of the order of action, [then] an entry into the realm of poetic composition, [and finally] a new configuration by means of this poetic refiguring of the pre-understood order of action" (p. xi). Thus we move from unconscious, the preunderstood, to the symbolically rendered conscious realm of subjective expression. It is compelling to note how this conception evokes comparison with Freud's (1900) topographical theory of consciousness, and how the conscious, preconscious, and unconscious systems interact.

For Ricoeur (1984), it is the mimetic function of plot that situates humans in time through the temporal values of action.

> What is ultimately at stake in the case of the structural identity of the narrative function as well as in that of the truth claim of every narrative work, is the temporal character of human experience. . . . Time becomes human time to the extent that it is organized after the manner of a narrative; narrative, in turn, is meaningful to the extent that it portrays the features of temporal experience. . . . [This is] a circular thesis, [but] a healthy circle, whose two halves mutually reinforce each other (p. 3).

Analysis of the narrative form of emplotted action, of experience that has been rendered symbolically, is an analysis of genre.

Frye's (1957) magisterial anatomy of literary genre provides some important guidelines for this endeavor. Based in myth, tragedy is the original form from which others develop. "Tragic drama derives from [the priestly performance of sacred ritual by] its central heroic figure, but the association of heroism with downfall is due to the simultaneous presence of irony. The nearer the tragedy is to [the sacred], the more closely associated the hero is to divinity; the nearer to irony, the more human the hero is, and the more the catastrophe appears to be a social rather than a cosmological event" (p. 284).

The presence of irony in a narrative strongly determines its formal character. The further comedy moves from irony, for example, the more lyrical it becomes. "The lyric reflects the sense of an external and social discipline" (p. 294) and thus is linked with how human beings fit into the cosmos. Lyric poetry from Horace to Hopkins to Whitman is devoted to this theme. Romance, the most lyric of dramatic forms, retains the ritual celebration of a natural order of humankind's relationship to nature after a challenge has disrupted that order, and has been set right. Shakespeare's last plays, *The Winter's Tale, Pericles,* and *The Tempest,* each show this progression from disorder to harmony. In satire, the form most heavily inflected with irony: "observation . . . is primary. . . . But as the observed phenomena move from the sinister to the grotesque, they grow more illusory and unsubstantial" (Frye, 1957, p. 298). Rabelais, Swift, and Voltaire used satire to launch bitter critiques of the commonplace social savagery they deplored in a manner more likely to engage their readers—fantastic fables. The Gothic narrative form that developed in the Romantic period has elements of both tragedy and satire. As Mary Shelley (1817) commented in *Frankenstein* on the ambitions of science as the age of empiricism dawned, the Gothic form is utterly free of the ironic diction of satire, while maintaining the ironic reversals of the tragic and often making observations on the culture from which it originated. The Gothic horror story is very closely linked with myth, as when the hero's downfall is inevitable because in his actions he has challenged divinity. The sinister observations are made in the interest of a cautionary moral lesson, but one that comes too late.

Two levels of abstraction, one focused on clusters of words and one on the level of genre, permit an approach to the material gathered in the interviews with my subjects. This approach illuminates what is specific to each of my coresearchers and provides insight as to the various constructions of meanings of being HIV-seropositive psychoanalysts. The theoretical perspective emanating from this theoretical synthesis and the analytic strategies associated with it animate an analysis that protects the identities of my coresearchers, relieves me of the awkward position of analyzing them, and also enables a means to make explicit what eludes language but is expressed symbolically through distinctly different formal narrative styles.

THREE NARRATIVE FORMS OF HIV SEROPOSITIVITY

My coresearchers' stories resemble three distinct genres: a romance in a lyrical mode, a satire in the style of the theatre of the absurd, and a Gothic tale of horror. In the romance, Coresearcher X underwent a series of trials, rather like Prince Tamino, the hero of Mozart and Schikaneder's (1791) *The Magic Flute*. Like Tamino, Coresearcher X experienced an ordeal by one of the three basic elements. The outcome has been a greater degree of insight and a conviction of a more genuine presence, so that the ordeal has made him more truly himself.

The absurdist satire's diction is predominantly ironic, and Coresearcher Y's narrative was heavily laden with an irony that expresses far more than words alone. The bitterest and most profound satire exposes our foolishness in thinking that our actions can possibly influence the world in which we live. As Esslin (1961) puts it, the absurdist writers express a "metaphysical anguish at the absurdity of the human condition" (pp. 23–24). Like Didi and Gogo in *Waiting for Godot* (Beckett, 1954), Y's narrative tells us that, although he knows he can't go on, he also knows that he has no choice *but* to go on. In the ironic satire, insight is helpful to us because it provides the necessary illusion that we are capable of doing something about life (about the HIV living inside us) *and* that this is an illusion. Some complain that Beckett's works are excessively nihilistic, but they overlook the courageous humanity of his hilariously benighted characters. "Didi and Gogo display steadfast faith and hope" (Esslin, 1961, p. 52). This is a narrative form that demands that we tolerate, indeed that we celebrate, paradox.

The Gothic narrative of Coresearcher Z describes the insight that comes about through the horrors visited on the subject coping with HIV disease. Like Bram Stoker's (1897) Count Dracula or Mary Shelley's (1817) Victor Frankenstein and his monstrous creation, Z experienced horrors that left him feeling isolated and forced him to learn lessons through an agonizing self-scrutiny. What is terrible is that this insight cannot stop further horrible events, nor does it provide a sense of connection with others. Insight is earned only through a solitary agony; sharing it is impossible. In the Gothic tale, the horrific action springs from the inability to face the limits of life and death, or, in a heroically definite idiom, the truth about our existence. Frankenstein is subtitled *The Modern Prometheus*, emphasizing the inevitable punishment for daring to challenge cosmic limits. Once we accept the necessarily solitary quality of the process of confronting and accepting these limits, we are on the way to attaining insight.

Eighty years later Stoker's *Dracula* (1897) elaborated themes appropriate to the era when Freud was beginning to analyze his first patients, hysterical young women. (Breuer's treatment of Anna O took place between 1880 and 1882; see Breuer and Freud, 1895.) Stoker's theme is the transgression of limits committed by perverse (or, according to some critics, female) sexuality (e.g., Stade, 1981; Craft, 1984; Hindle, 1993). If we do not accept these limitations, we are destroyed, or transformed into monsters, as the victims of Frankenstein and Dracula learn. That there is this goal at the end allows us to note the heroic contour of the Gothic narrative: a building climax that culminates in a resolution. This resolution often has about it the sense of renunciation of our former illusions, made possible by the reversal of fortune that characterizes the tragic form.

These narrative forms are expressed in the stories told on several themes determined by my questions through the interviews: on being HIV positive, on HIV as an identity, the clinical context, the question of disclosure, and the analyst's fears and disappointments. More general themes are articulated as well, such as dependence–autonomy, passivity –activity, and sameness–difference. These themes, valences in anyone's personality style rather than specific to a particular condition, are axes upon which experiences and attendant meanings of HIV/AIDS turn, playing out a range of variations.

THE NARRATIVE OF LYRICAL ROMANCE

Coresearcher X's story of being HIV positive is dominated by certain clusters of words. Describing the time after he first tested positive, he repeats the phrase "examining my body" and notes that he felt "obsessive" until there was a "shift." He sets up a dichotomy between a relationship with the doctor that is "based on fear" and "fear driven" and an approach that is more "holistic," more "Eastern," and so "more positive" and "more empowering." The story at this point is the conflict between an approach to his HIV status that is "based on fear" and one based on "empowerment." Through "a long process" he is able to "accept this situation." With the importance of acceptance we note the presence of "one initiative of lyric . . . [that] corresponds to . . . the epiphany in drama" (Frye, 1957, p. 293). He rejects an approach to medical care that seems "fear driven" to him and feels confident enough to disagree with his physician when the doctor suggests starting medication, such as early intervention with AZT when this was thought to be the best way to treat HIV infection.

The story of attaining his self-acceptance begins to emerge when certain words and phrases, and the order and contiguity in which they occur, are attended to. Clusters of words like "kill it" and "kill parts of myself" are repeated. These come in the context of what he *didn't* have to do, but a heroic struggle is going on, nonetheless. After these clusters of "kill it" and "kill parts of myself," X uses the phrases "self-acceptance and love" and "the best path." Like Tamino slaying the dragon, the opening event of Mozart's (1791) opera *The Magic Flute*, his journey toward insight is begun.

The process that X describes has to do with arriving at a point of view about his health that emphasizes his autonomy and strength. Many of his remarks seem to express his determination to see things in an optimistic light, such as "health," "a healthy lifestyle," "things I do to take care of myself," and "I keep in mind that I am healthy," which clearly indicate this intention. The other emotional valence is expressed in phrases such as "pangs of anxiety," "fear-driven," "driven by dependencies," and "waiting to get sick." It seems to be dependence and passivity that X confronts and must overcome. When the story progresses to the point where he has achieved this task, the clusters of words repeated most often are "health," "healthy," "self-acceptance," and "healing." The culmination emphasizes his achievement of a sense of empowerment and autonomy.

Part of the process of achieving this empowerment is a transformation of identity. X asserts that HIV seropositivity constitutes a substantial aspect of a person's identity, and that being genuine means embracing this aspect of himself. He repeats statements such as "That's who I am today" and "It's part of who I am." He uses words such as "comfortable" and "natural" when describing this sense of HIV and identity. In the three narratives under discussion here, only X's places this generative value on being HIV positive as an identity.

In the clinical context, though, X's adjustments that enabled him to maintain his optimistic point of view seem more vulnerable to question. There are difficulties that arise while listening to material that is fraught with anxiety and pain, that evoke memories of HIV-related events he has lived through. Though he acknowledges that analysts and patients may be more the same than different, particularly when confronting fears associated with catastrophic illness, it has often been necessary to regard himself as not sick, not like his patients. He uses a sort of spontaneous hierarchy of HIV illness in which ascending positions on a scale define a difference that seems to help in maintaining the adaptive denial that makes it possible to continue being a therapist.

At this point, he describes how the battle between fear and empowerment begins again: "There's me, and there's the other. He finds that he must maintain a certain healthy denial or dissociation in order to maintain his sense of empowerment. But in this battle, he also finds the benefit of confronting the realities of the illness, and this prevents him from avoiding facing his fears. It is just this confrontation, in his daily clinical work, that reinforces his stance of seeing himself as positive and healthy. With the outcome of this confrontation between fear and empowerment, responsibility and autonomy are (once again) the most highly valued virtues.

On disclosure, Coresearcher X describes a "natural" process during which his HIV status "comes out." It has to do with honor, with respect, and with being genuine. For him, it is a question neither of disclosing nor denying, but simply an inevitable part of an unfolding relationship with a patient. This relationship involves being brave and having respect. Technically, however, his approach to answering direct questions from patients continues to include exploration "to get to the essence" of what they want to know. This sense of getting to the essence is consonant with his experience of HIV assuming a substantial meaning in his identity, that there is an essential truth to be located.

An essence that is uncovered also repeats a theme crucial to the form of the romance, where the protagonist's journey, or process, culminates in the achievement of maturity and insight. Romance's "idealizing of heroism and purity" lends it a tendency toward allegory (Frye, 1957, p. 306), an inflection apparent here. In perhaps the most affect-laden portion of X's narrative, he elaborates his most urgent confrontation with fear. This event assumes the pivotal point in the story. In a trial by water (in the form of scuba-diving lessons), he must live through a great terror, of "going down," of "crawling on the bottom" and facing his "fear of life and death." Finally daring to go under the water, he acknowledges his own vulnerability, his own mortality. Difference and sameness oscillate, setting up a potentially confusing situation as he experiences what he assumes some of his phobic patients experience. Surviving the ordeal gives him a new appreciation for all kinds of fears and phobias. Survival also means that his autonomy and empowerment have been reestablished and consolidated.

Structurally, the episode of the trial by water marks a climax that is followed by events describing the consolidation of his role as a mature analyst. Here he engages in a battle with an idealized internal analyst figure, someone who ought to be an "expert," a state he acknowledges he will not live up to. Belonging to two social groups (gay men and psychoanalysts), he experiences a further tension. The theme of stigma becomes prominent and requires management. At this point in the narrative structure, survival of the stigmatic identification becomes a further test to endure.

As he speaks about his sense of the stigma attached to HIV seropositivity within the analytic community, the linkage between HIV/AIDS and gay men emerges. The challenge resides in confronting this interpretive link made by others, particularly colleagues in the field of psychoanalysis. Noteworthy, too, is the conjunction of being a gay man who is HIV positive: that it connotes promiscuity, having been or being a "party boy." This equation, dating to the earliest days of life with HIV/AIDS, is so durable as to dominate X's sense of his reception by his colleagues in 1999.

For Coresearcher X, his HIV status and his sexual orientation function not so much as markers but as substantive aspects of a self that can be hidden or revealed. But he describes the effects of revealing these aspects of himself as promoting the dismantling of stigma. He refers at this point to the stronger presence of openly gay analysts in recent years, which suggests that it is not the content, but the very act of exchange that is transformative, that it is the doing battle that is crucial. The transformation may be benevolent, in a clinical situation, or it may be potentially destructive, in a collegial situation where his professional identity may be called into question.

In the course of this battle, he sets forth his theoretical approach in detail: how this departs in some way from traditional technique, and why he believes it is important to do so. Because of the kinds of experiences he's "grappled," "gone to war," and "battled it out with," he has something special he can offer in his work. He has earned the right to think independently. Perhaps more important, though, is his sense that he has a responsibility to offer this part of himself to others. This part of the story, then, marks a culmination of the protagonist's tests, the demonstration of his readiness to assume the station he's earned. All that remains is the ceremonial acknowledgment of this achievement.

The final chapter of X's romance is the description of such a ceremony. He has been called upon to play an important role, to be witnessed by several generations of family and colleagues. This event, positioned at the end of X's narrative, performs the same structural functions as the wedding of Tamino to Pamina at the end of *The Magic Flute*, or of Florizel to Perdita at the end of *The Winter's Tale*. In the romance, these ceremonials mark the restoration of a "natural" order, along with the marking of the protagonist's assumption of a position of maturity and insight. X's participation in a public ceremony, involving speaking before a large group, performs a similar structural function, establishing his importance in his chosen role, having battled with the fears associated with his HIV-positive status and surviving tests demonstrating his maturity, autonomy, and empowerment.

That he could survive these tests seems explicitly connected to his theoretical and technical approach to treatment, where a process of mutual involvement is seen as curative. This sense of the benefits of mutuality holds true for his relationships beyond the treatment situation. X describes an evolving sense of his HIV status and how this aspect of his identity relates to his role as an analyst and to the analytic community. The most important values throughout the narrative of the lyrical romance have been connection, respect, understanding, and mutuality. Although there is a conviction that X's HIV seropositivity has a substantial quality (as if it determines an identity), it is the performative aspect of doing battle with the associated fears of this identity, and disclosing this detail of his life, that effects changes in relationships with others.

THE NARRATIVE OF ABSURDIST SATIRE

Like the blasted landscapes of Beckett's plays, where location is defined more by what it is not than by any distinctive traits, Coresearcher Y's narrative is dominated by negations. On being HIV positive, for example, he "never thinks about it," it is "not part of [his] sense of identity," he's "able to block it out." These phrases are uttered with a deadpan delivery, expressing an ambivalence that eventually becomes explicit. Although he never thinks about being HIV positive, there are two stark possibilities for the future: either he'll get "a shot" and he'll be cured, or there will be "a major stock market crash, or World War III" and manufacture of medicines will cease, and he'll "die of AIDS." But once these possibilities are spelled out, the ironically inflected negations take over: HIV is "not even a backdrop," it is "inconsequential," "not on my mind," and the word "never" is repeated, over and over again. All of this is delivered with a rather comic, knowing style that signals the listener to assume that intense feelings are wrapped up inside the ironic exterior. Although HIV is negated, not affecting his "personality" and "disowned," he also describes himself as explosive with an anger that seemed inevitable but does not require any explanation. It is as if he says both "How could anyone dream of *not* being angry?" and "Isn't this hilarious?"

Esslin (1961), writing about the theatre of the absurd, argues that "the form, structure, and mood of an artistic statement cannot be separated from its meaning, its conceptual content; simply because the work of art as a whole *is* its meaning, *what* is said in it is indissolubly linked with the *manner* in which it is said, and cannot be said in any other way" (p. 44). Psychoanalytic therapists' clinical experience would most assuredly confirm this point of view. Feelings in the narrative of the absurdist satire are disparate, expressed glibly in a style that makes it impossible for the content not to be understood in multiple ways. Y's glib, straightforward delivery acknowledges the presence of feelings, particularly anger, and is often bitterly funny. Packed within each admission is a double negation: this is what I *don't* feel, which of course indicates that it *is felt* and isn't it *funny* that I am saying that I don't feel anything, because we both know that I *am*, in fact, feeling this, and how could this *actually* be funny. This complex structure imparts to each episode of the narrative (what it was like to learn of his HIV seropositivity, how it never affects his work, how he approaches his work, and that he never tells anyone about it) another doubleness: that however much insight we may be able to acquire, natural forces like viruses will remain implacably beyond our control.

In the clinical context, Y describes "never missing a day" of work, even if he has a fever due to side effects of medication. Again this is related in the form of a comic story: how ridiculous he is to work through this condition, and how absurd it is that none of his patients have noticed anything different about him. The ironically disowned aspect of this story is that he is able to go on working no matter what, even when he feels as if he can't. Coresearcher Y's narrative depends on this doubleness of structure. And in his satiric diction, he echoes Estragon and Vladimir in Beckett's (1954) *Waiting for Godot:* "I can't go on like this." "That's what you think" (p. 109). The absurdist satire invites us to share in the joke that is always on ourselves.

The satiric quality of Y's story fades as he describes his clinical work. He is concerned that the needs of his patients must remain always in the foreground, and to that end, his style of negating his condition is consonant with this goal. This dedication is told in an episode that includes a gently self-mocking admission of his own wishes, maintaining the structural form of the satire but communicating clearly the extreme seriousness of his approach.

Y relates how he never tells anyone about being HIV positive, that he rarely discloses anything. But in the next moment, he asserts that he would disclose if he were HIV negative. This swift oscillation between extremes, a comic device that works to keep both sides of a question open even as, on the surface, it denies both, is the means whereby both sides of the themes of autonomy–dependence, activity–passivity, and sameness–difference are kept in play. HIV is immaterial, but if he were negative his status *would* be disclosed. By not thinking about HIV, he remains autonomous, not defining himself according to a medical condition, but in this admission is an acknowledgement that he will also always be dependent on his strategy of remaining "guarded." Through his action of working without pause, without allowing for interruptions due to his condition, there is the implied acknowledgment that he'd be swamped by passivity if he did stop. If he told others about his HIV serostatus, he'd be the same as a group he is contemptuous of, those who "make HIV a cause" or "put it at the forefront" of their identity, and irrevocably different from those who are free of the virus.

Fears of the future are handled in the same manner. He "wouldn't be surprised if there was a 100 percent cure," and he "wouldn't be surprised if HIV killed me." He does not rule out that his medications may cause "cancer, diabetes, blood clots, or a heart attack" and "kill me." Even as he tells me he's "very fatalistic," he can imagine a time when it will have been helpful to have faced a terminal illness and lived, because that may attract potential patients. Fatalism is inflected with an ironic admission of planning for the future, which is accompanied by an admission of feeling ashamed for doing so.

The doubleness that inflects Y's planning for the future emphasizes a problem for HIV-positive individuals in what Rofes (1998) has termed "the protease moment" (p. 29). Now that it is more possible than ever to consider HIV a chronically manageable condition (for those who respond optimally to the new medications), we are faced with a very particular experience of the passage of time. We wait for the next generation of medications or for our health to finally begin to deteriorate, with the knowledge of the continual flux caused by the life of the virus inside us. Here is another point of convergence with the absurdist satire enacted by Beckett's tramps. "Waiting is to experience the action of time, which is constant change" (Esslin, 1961, p. 52). And here we confront "the problem of the nature of the self, which, being subject to constant change in time, is in constant flux and therefore ever outside our grasp. . . . We're always not identical with ourselves" (pp. 50–51). As Beckett's everymen wait, experiencing the constant change of time, nothing really happens. "And yet, as nothing real ever happens, that change is in itself an illusion. The ceaseless activity of time is self-defeating, purposeless, and therefore null and void," but despite all of this, Didi and Gogo live in hope (Esslin, 1961, pp. 50–51). Or like Winnie, the heroine of Beckett's (1961) *Happy Days*, who, although buried up to her neck, Esslin (1961) sees as maintaining a "cheerfulness in the face of death and nothingness [that] is an expression of man's courage and nobility. . . . Winnie's life does consist of happy days, because she refuses to be dismayed" (p. 83). This, finally, is the most important aspect of the absurdist narrative as exemplified in Beckett's characters: that we go on, despite ourselves, courageously living in hope.

By emplotting the story of his HIV seropositivity in the satiric absurd, Coresearcher Y is able to express and keep open at least two sides to each question. This formal structure reveals what is most important to know about the content of this narrative of being HIV positive and working as an analyst (perhaps more to the point, about working as an analyst at all), that everything is always both/and. He can't go on, and he'll go on. Like Winnie in *Happy Days*, he'll greet the day cheerfully, attending fully to all the necessary, insignificant details of another day.

THE NARRATIVE OF GOTHIC HORROR

Coresearcher Z's narrative begins with the phrase "a death sentence." Immediately, we are plunged into a frightening world where everything seems "useless" and things "make no sense." The details and even the temporal order of events are difficult for the narrator to keep straight. Things feel uncanny. Things are "blurry" and it is all too easy to "forget." Yet HIV and the ensuing events made necessary by some troubling physical symptoms are "always there." The atmosphere is murky, terror-filled, and both forgotten and unforgettable. The specter of impending death renders him "distracted," full of "fear," and "anxious." His "mind is always somewhere else." These repeated verbal fragments and the structuring of the narrative beginning with a "death sentence" evoke an atmosphere of Gothic horror.

Once this climate of dread is established, clusters of words comprising two narrative strains that become almost character-like emerge in Z's story. One is the objective scientist of the empirical ideal, the scientist who probes what is to be observed closely and who always needs to go further in that probing. Feelings are suspect and must be held in check. Needs, his own in particular, are to be scrutinized. The scientist must always ask, "What kind of need?" or "What is the nature of that need?" This voice observes that he is "not thinking clearly" and deplores that he did "a very bad thing" and "makes mistakes." Clarity and a detached objectivity are values important to this character in the story. The scientist is also a strict moralist who deplores his own tendency to see "HIV as a grand excuse for everything."

The other character is prone to strong feelings of "envy," "jealousy," "anger," and "bitterness," affects that are repeatedly named. This voice can describe the "terrible burden" and "awful fears" that come with HIV seropositivity. In some ways, this character, prone to uncontrollable affects, takes on traits of often pathetic, victimized, and victimizing figures of Gothic horror who are doomed to a solitary existence, most familiarly Frankenstein's creature, or Dracula. What could be more monstrous for a therapist than finding limits to her or his capacity for empathy? For this character, the idea of watching another get sicker, "slowly deteriorating," signals another immersion into horror. At this point in the narration, Z admits that this is a "constant reminder of the frightening thing," that "disturbing, frightening thing" that is "always there" but that usually he "blocks out."

The establishment of these two characters sets up a mysterious conflict between "two opposing forces," between the objective scientist fighting to maintain his observing stance and something that threatens to take him over. This other is the monstrous creature of HIV, "disrupting," "erupting," with a "need, a pressing need" that will "interfere" and render him unable to be a therapist. This conflict echoes the structure of Shelley's (1816) *Frankenstein*, which, as Stark (1951) argued, is about two opposing aspects of a single person. Johnson (1991) observes that "the scenes of his [Victor Frankenstein's] daring experiment are conducted, appropriately, at the top of the house, in an attic, metaphor of derangement or misguided intellectual pursuit" (p. xii). This metaphor also reinforces the notion that the conflict unfolds within one consciousness.

We learn more about how Coresearcher Z's conflict was set in motion through an episode related to painful and invasive medical treatments that was "horrible . . . horrible beyond belief." It caused a "dramatic change" and left him on one side of "a divide" where there is "no one left." The narrator recalls this dreadful sequence fitfully; at moments he "can't remember" (he is "good at blocking"), then worries about the effect his recounting of it will have on his audience. Indeed, the effect this does have is to deepen the sense of horror, of mystery, echoing a device familiar to those who have heard ghost stories told late at night. This is in no way to suggest that Z is consciously using a narrative device, but to point out a formal similarity between his story and the structure of the Gothic horror tale, both of which often use epistolary framing devices to interrupt the narrative flow and allow direct authorial address to the reader.

Surviving the horrible experience leaves the hero transformed, chastened. Now that "it's over" and "it's part of history," he is "toughened up." On the other side of a "divide," he has become aware that now it is "hard to listen" to a story like his experience of horror. He "doesn't want to listen" and feels that although he "knows what it is like" to undergo such awful things, still it "goes against the grain" to listen. Having "done battle" with the horror, his conviction is that others, too, must become able to "tough it out." Knowledge of this kind of horror only seems attainable by doing battle alone, in isolation, like Harker's journey to Dracula's castle in Transylvania, or Victor Frankenstein's fight to the death with his terrible creation on fields of ice.

The words fear, fearful, agony, and murky set the tone for this portion of the narrative, functioning as, in words that are repeated often, "careful . . . reminders." The Gothic is nothing if not a cautionary tale, warning the uninitiated away from going too far into the dark. Coresearcher Z reminds himself of the perils of going into the dark again, too; that HIV, though it "is always there" and "permeates everything," can be "overplayed"—that is, he runs the risk of giving way to a kind of weakness that has eaten away at him.

Decaying transformation such as that in a Gothic narrative like Poe's (1845) *The Fall of the House of Usher*, repeats the action of a gradual but implacable destruction of the immune system that is the action of HIV. It is expressed in diction as well as structure. The presence of malevolent metamorphosis at the level of the sentence is announced through the repetition of words in Z's story such as shift, shifting, eruption, disruption, deteriorating, and, perhaps most salient, permeates. Just as horror permeates the atmosphere of the Gothic tale, infection permeates the body of the HIV-positive person. (Francis Ford Coppola's 1992 film version of *Dracula*, made when the AIDS crisis was at its apogee in the United States, emphasizes the life-sustaining power of blood that is perverted by the vampire's need. It depicts a frightening transformation that takes place in the blood of the vampire's victim.) In imagination, this physical transformation can be expressed through the structuring of the narrative in a form that repeats the action of soaking in horror until everything is tainted with it. All these examples of the Gothic genre—from Poe, Stoker, and even Shelley—have a seroconversion and its repercussions type of theme. Once he is tainted by an abhorrent but fascinating transgression of natural laws, the protagonist becomes dangerous to others. He is infectious. The contagion must be contained and killed. The Gothic is pessimistic about the secrets lurking within or behind the natural world and the relationship of human beings with those secrets.

It is especially noteworthy that a conflictual relationship to the cosmos and the cautionary moral message that is so intrinsic to the Gothic narrative have been elaborated in the way HIV has been understood as the natural result of perverse and sinful actions. Shelley's (1861) *Frankenstein* has been described as an implicit reading of Milton's *Paradise Lost* (Bloom, 1965, p. 214), or a subversion of that epic poem (Steiner, 1999). Here the allegory is of the fall from grace and the expulsion from the garden. Stoker's (1897) *Dracula*, too, has been described as a Christian allegory, with its central metaphor being the exchange of blood (Wolf, 1992, p. viii). True to the period of its composition (the beginning of the Freudian era), sexuality is highlighted in *Dracula*, even a suppressed homoeroticism, in the estimation of one critic. According to this reading, the novel's primary anxiety "derives from Dracula's hovering interest in Jonathan Harker. . . . [A sexual threat that the novel] first evokes, manipulates, sustains, but never finally represents is that Dracula will seduce, penetrate, drain another male" (Craft, 1984, pp. 109–110). The specter of homosexuality, so intrinsic to the story of HIV, is detected in Stoker's tale. These themes have been enacted, repeated, between the two characterized aspects of himself that emerged in Coresearcher Z's narrative. The action, the mimesis carried out by his story's emplotment, works in two directions. His story expresses frightening personal feelings and experiences, moving from within the individual toward others and also expressing the moral attitudes that echo those emanating from a collective point of view toward the individual, censuring, warning, and punishing. The structure and diction of the Gothic tale elaborates horrors and their lessons, moving toward a resolution that is not an assurance of safety, but a warning to be vigilant. As Z's narrative demonstrates, the Gothic tale effectively expresses, even anticipates, much of the history of HIV's narrative emplotment.

NARRATIVE FORM, MIMESIS, AND REPETITION

For the coresearchers, HIV-positive serostatus has been a medium in which crucial aspects of their experience have been structured in distinctive ways. These three widely divergent narrative forms, which carry meaning effects in their very structure, reveal a range of affective relationships to HIV seropositivity. The lyric romance describes a progressive movement toward an intersubjective paradise, where a refiner's fire makes the hero more like himself than he's ever been before. Confronting the meanings of HIV seropositivity, particularly in the context of doing psychoanalytic work, is rendered as a quest that ends in triumph commemorated by a public recognition. The absurdist satire argues that nothing can possibly be so neat and that triumphs are illusions—the most we can hope for is the capacity to laugh ironically as we continue our hapless struggle. Paradox is the defining structural element of the satire, carrying a crucial meaning effect that pertains to HIV: that we are sick, and that we are not sick. The form of the Gothic tale of horror is weighted toward pessimism, cautioning us against the monstrous needs and feelings that hide in dark recesses along with the virus. The moral lesson that is central to the Gothic narrative, that challenges to the cosmological order will be punished, has been repeated in the narrative emplotment of HIV, as well: it is a divine retribution for perversion and sin.

HIV set in motion stories that, in their dialogic unfolding, took on forms, plots. The dialogic unfolding did not end when our interviews were over but continued as I repeated, in dialogue with myself, these stories. It was through this repetition that the forms, the plots, became clear to me, in a process evocative of the transformation of unformulated experience into that which can be imagined and *used* (Stern, 1997). This analysis has defined more clearly three disparate fantasies associated with HIV seropositivity, fantasies that, it seems to me, must be heard in concert with each other. It is important to preserve all these constructed meanings, with their contradictory, complementary and ameliorative aspects intact, in the interest of beginning to express as much nuance and detail of the overwhelming multiplicity of an experience of HIV seropositivity as can be uttered at a given point in time.

This formal analysis of the stories of HIV seropositivity reveals an aspect of the general question of disclosure that tends to be neglected, and that is the narrative form in which a disclosure might be emplotted. Although disclosures have often been discussed as if they were reports of facts about the analyst, they are also stories that are told in a certain way. The fact described in a report may impart far less than the narrative style in which it is told, revealing something about how the teller organizes her or his experience.[1]

But this formal analysis suggests another general proposition: that the repetitions of these forms stretch backward in time, before these interviews as well, before we knew HIV, even. Each coresearcher's experience of HIV seropositivity found an emplotment through an imagined mimesis of the preunderstood through the action of telling, of repeating, in order to move what was on the threshold of consciousness into the realm of the symbolic and thus the knowable. It is through the telling that what was poised at the edge of understanding is transformed into a kind of action that makes meaning possible. Put in the most radical way, a knowing comes about through a doing. This knowing about the meanings

---

[1] I am indebted to John Kerr for pointing out this generalizable theme.

of being an HIV-positive psychoanalyst came about through telling stories that carried meaning effects in their narrative structure as well as in the specific content. It was through repetition, in intersubjective space, that the meaning effects carried in narrative forms could be lived in the telling and registered with another.

CHAPTER 6

AN ANALYST PREPARES

IN THE YEARS THAT HAVE passed since I began thinking about this project, my relationships to psychoanalysis and to HIV have changed. It is probably more accurate to say that these are constantly changing. The preceding chapters detail how I felt that certain changes in my clinical practice were necessitated by my HIV status, a status that is in constant flux. Often, changes in my relationship to the virus are prompted by readings of T-cell counts and viral activity. In response to these changes, I have started more than one medication regime, stopped one in order to see whether or not it was doing anything, been alarmed at the speed with which viral activity skyrocketed in my blood, and started a new one. Sometimes the relationship changes in response to those moments when my serostatus is foregrounded because of the risk of exposing another to one of my body fluids—my infectious potential must be accounted for in some way. Other moments are marked by a change that is not anchored in the actual at all, when desire or memory awakens an imaginative link with some aspect of HIV seropositivity. At times it has seemed like an open question whether I have made these changes or whether these changes have made me. It is a stormy relationship, quiet for a time, sometimes demanding attention. This final chapter is an attempt to find a way into this knot, a way to think more clearly about what has happened in my clinical work and in my private experience.

Several years ago the protease inhibitors changed the trajectory of HIV infection for a great many HIV-positive people. We had organized ourselves around one narrative of HIV progression and were granted the luxury (or the curse) of inventing a new narrative for ourselves. Some lived through a dramatic Lazarus syndrome, when the protease inhibitors literally raised them from their deathbeds. Others, like me, were lucky enough to have these new medications in time to defer any palpable signs of HIV illness. Now we find ourselves trusting optimistically that newer generations of medicine will become available to avert illness again and again. With this proviso, I can now envision the expectable and comforting insults that encroaching middle age brings, rather than edgily anticipating one or two drastic infections that would cut my life short.

As I worked through recollections of my work with Kent, Jasper, and Jack, my seropositivity brought into stark contrast certain ideals and fantasies that partly determined the course of clinical moments I encountered, despite my stable health supported by the effective medications. My idealizations of the role of psychoanalyst, for example, complicated the process of thinking through decisions as to how to begin and to conduct treatments with certain patients. These idealizations worked in the service of establishing and maintaining a sense of professional identity, one that sometimes felt consonant with a private identity, and at other times felt confining and dissonant. By examining how these idealizations were formed and how they are supported (perhaps even engendered) by aspects of a psychoanalytic culture, I have been able to work more freely and openly. Yet I still wish to find ways to describe an identity that functions as a process rather than as a construction in which I am living.

Barthes (1977) describes:

> A frequent image . . . the *Argo* (luminous and white), each piece of which the Argonauts gradually replaced, so that they ended with an entirely new ship, without having to alter either its name or its form. This ship *Argo* is highly useful; it affords the allegory of an eminently structural object, created not by genius, inspiration, determination, evolution, but by two modest actions (which cannot be caught up in any mystique of creation): *substitution* (one part replaces another, as in a paradigm) and *nomination* (the name is in no way linked to the stability of the parts): by dint of

combinations made within one and the same name, nothing is left of the *origin: Argo* is an object with no other cause
than its name, with no other identity than its form [p. 46].

This image conveys a great deal about a different way to experience oneself, about what a psychoanalytic treatment can offer, and
about how it makes that offer. Substitution is one of the mecha-
nisms by which psychoanalysis claims to understand and interpret
the speech of the unconscious. It is also the key to the analyst's role:
the analyst is a substitute, but the real thing, too. Nomination is
calling oneself into being as the role assigned, or having that role
assigned by another. An original that has been revised (through
combinations of the new) continues to be called by the old name.

Barthes's image also reminded me of an article I read some years
ago about the hopes for eradicating HIV from the body, from which
I learned that every cell of our bodies is replaced over a period of
five to seven years. This article put forth the theory that, once it
was possible to suppress the level of virus sufficiently, this process
of gradual replacement of cells could eventually leave the body free
of any trace of HIV. It would be rather like having all one's timbers
replaced in the course of a long, epic adventure, having left an unde-
sirable crewmember on a deserted island along the way (like another
seagoing Greek, Philoctetes, who was put ashore by Odysseus owing
to his putrifying wound). Unfortunately, Odysseus found to his
consternation that he needed Philoctetes and his bow after all. And
we, to ours, are finding that the virus is not so easy to abandon.

HIV, with its profusion of meanings, seems to inspire this kind
of avid speculation. In this imaginary way it functions like what
Derrida (1978) calls "supplement" (p. 199). That is, HIV has become
a vivid example of how we manipulate a metaphor to make of the
known an allusion to the unknown. But the metaphor of HIV is
also a great example of how metaphors manipulate us. This is evi-
dent not only in the response of the uninfected to those carrying
the virus, but also in the formation of identities founded on being
HIV positive. As many have pointed out, the lushly proliferating
meanings surrounding HIV are all too familiar: transgression, mon-
strosity, evil, death (e.g., Treichler, 1988). Certain kinds of sex

become metaphors and gay men are transformed into irresponsible libertines carrying contagion that threatens untold numbers of innocent victims. HIV mutates in the imagination as well as in the body, resisting a reified knowing. Trying to think about HIV/AIDS, we focus on these constructed meanings of the syndrome and see that HIV is yet another iteration of our approach toward the limit of the unknown. Our rehearsal of familiar metaphors, and possibly of innovative ones, is all that is possible. I may think that I have come to understand something substantive about what the virus means, but once I think that, I've lost what is far more important: the action of the virus. When HIV enters a healthy blood cell, a transformation occurs, a kind of mutation, as a previously benign blood cell becomes a carrier of HIV. This process has a location and a substance, which makes thinking of difference easier. But the action of mutation, of difference, is an event, not a substance. The action of mutation is where difference happens, and even in that phrase I am tempted to assign a location for difference, already implying a substance. But that is an illusion. The task is to attend to the action of approaching the limits of what can be known.

And so we keep at it, approaching the threshold of the unknown. In the many ways that the experience of managing stigmatized identities has been explicated, the problem of difference as difference keeps forcing itself upon our attention. Our conceptions of different or deviant identities often function within a paradigm where the relationship between the normal and the deviant is understood to be dialectical and context specific, and where either party can play both parts. Difference is then unmasked as constructed from identity. Difference is known through action, whether that action takes place in the mind or in social encounters. It is a mimetic relationship, rather than one that is available to a direct knowledge of essences. Often in the enactment that depends on and reveals difference, social roles are revealed to be metaphoric masks that correspond, with varying degrees of authenticity, to an inner life. And as some of my coresearchers' remarks suggested, stigma could even determine a relationship between two members within the stigmatized group of the HIV-positive. Contact with difference will require that we pay attention to what is strategically enacted.

Difference and Dissociation

Freud's great challenge was the notion that a radical, unknowable difference resides within us all: the unconscious. We infer it only through derivatives that become knowable through processes such as metaphor and metonymy, allowing us—sometimes forcing us— to speak in spite of ourselves. Hints of the action of difference become traceable in clinical process at work as bits of retrospective awareness that are among the more gratifying moments in a psychoanalytic treatment, when what has been dissociated becomes knowable. It is that moment when we can almost feel the transformation of a bit of unformulated experience (Stern, 1997) into a knowable form.

Dissociations become available to our knowing in a large range of ways. My colleagues emplotted their experiences of HIV seropositivity as a means of encoding aspects of dissociated experience. Coming to understand the content expressed in certain formal traits, such as the genre or dramatic structure of their stories, enables us to notice what eludes conscious awareness. Classically, dreams and waking fantasies provide another means of access to the dissociated. Kent and I experienced this in the moment when he discovered a fantasy creation, expressed in the recovery of his recurring dream, that exerted a wonderful explanatory effect. Still another means of knowing dissociated aspects of oneself is through the retrospective analysis of what has been enacted. The contents of Kent's fantasy, that he was buried alive with the father whom he'd hoped would rescue him, had cast an enormous influence over his relationships. An enactment of the scenario, including his affective experience of despair, had unfolded in his relationship with me, as well as in his life beyond our work.

The dissociated content of emplotment and enactment becomes knowable through action that has assumed a dramatic form, a mimetic repetition occurring in the space between people. We must play it in order to know it. Once, psychoanalysis deemed enactments to be detrimental to the clinical progress—acting out had to be avoided. Now, it is the ubiquity of enactment that is often acknowledged as the very means by which to reach transforming understanding. We enact through our bodies; indeed, we are able to enact because we have bodies. To accommodate the importance of embodied action, the concept of transference has been expanded to provide a context for understanding the physical aspects of the drama as well as imagined relationships between therapist and patient.

For example, Harris (1998) prepares the way for a relational theory of the body, a "view of body states and processes as inseparable from fantasy, interaction, and meaning" (p. 43). For Harris, meaning must encompass "a range of representations of experience: linguistic, symbolic, imagistic, perceptual" (p. 44). This, Harris argues, is continuous with Freud's vision of the ego as "a body ego" or "a psychic manifestation of a corporeal projection" (p. 42). Although body states and processes are inseparable from meaning, these two registers of experience are not entirely overlapping. Our physical experience escapes symbolization and entrance into what is knowable, and at the same time no bodily experience can be known outside our symbolized ways of knowing. It is as if our bodies "behave us," and it is afterward, by attempting to represent this experience to ourselves, that we can know about it. We become aware of what is included, as well as what escapes from our experience, because we are embedded in the context of social interactions, which are bounded by time and space. That is, Harris points out, it is the experience of being a body among bodies that gives rise to psychic experience. That much of bodily experience escapes our knowing lends a sense of effervescence to a description of psychic life, as if we are constantly in the process of coming into being. What anchors us in time is the bodily action of mimesis (the process through which we come to represent ourselves to ourselves), and language (how we speak ourselves to ourselves).

Harris (1998) writes:

> Mimesis, the experience of merging self in the experience of the other, is an experience both active and passive, creating body ego through a use or appropriation of the other, but an other who is an active seer and constructor, not a neutral feedback apparatus. From the charged social interplay in which self–other distinctions are blurred and dissolving, body ego

and psychic identity thus emerge as inextricably social and also psychic. Mimesis is an experience in which spatial distinctiveness collapses in an experience of being the other [p. 46].

Harris describes an experience of merging with another. But I would add that this is a process in which limits are also discovered, through their abrogation. Eventually the mimetic process also involves the reestablishment of sharp edges in a dialectical fashion. The appropriation of the other is an encounter with an active constructor, an other who exerts an effect, leaves an imprint, on the subject. There must be something there to be constructed, on which to register. For all the dissolving, there is also a coming into being of the self through Harris's description of a mimetic process. Spatial distinctiveness collapses but then reintegrates with borders.

Just as bodily experience can be understood as involving a complex interaction of merging and finding edges, so language serves a similar function. Ricoeur (1992) details a description of the ways our use of language provides us with a sense of being anchored in time, and so knowable to ourselves. But he argues that what we come to know is not a substantial essence, a self as a thing, but a limit, another kind of border. Ricoeur uses the word identical in a way that has two meanings. It is "at the center of our reflections on personal identity and narrative identity and related to a primary trait of the self, namely its temporality" (p. 2). By this he urges us to remember that the term identity functions both as an instance and as a continuity in time. But identity ought not to be understood as implying something that does not change over time. Not only is identity continuous and changing, but Ricoeur "suggests from the outset that the selfhood of oneself implies otherness to such an intimate degree that one cannot be thought of without the other, that instead one passes into the other." (p. 3). He posits a merging, one that is revealed and that occurs through a speech practice that establishes a sense of limit.

In Ricoeur's linguistic analysis, what anchors a self, what enables the sense of identity, is practice—that is, the way we go about in the world by acting in and upon it: how we *do* things. Thus speech, "the act of speaking itself, which designates the speaker reflexively. Pragmatics, therefore, puts directly on stage the 'I' and the 'you' of the speech situation" (p. 40). But once the stage is set for a pragmatic demonstration of self as identical to itself, Ricoeur argues that an I is not to be taken as more than a place marker, a token. He points out that our speech practice seems to disguise what relational psychoanalysts know: that there is no such thing as an isolated "I." "Indeed, what sense are we to attach to the idea of a *singular perspective* on the world?" (p. 51). When we think we occupy a singular perspective, or what amounts to "the privileged point of perspective on the world which each speaking subject is," what we encounter is "the limit of the world and not one of its contents" (p. 51). We find ourselves at a boundary.

The self is seen to be a discrete subject when a limit is encountered, as the infant encounters the limit of his or her absolute self (Benjamin, 1988), or as we notice some slip of the tongue, thereby encountering a limit mark of what we confidently know about ourselves. It is the play of these edges, and the extent to which we can appreciate them, from which emanates an important valence of our experience of identity.

Mimesis, stage, enact, role: the words we use to gain understanding of certain unconscious processes depend on a theatrical metaphor of actors playing out a drama on a stage that seems both psychic and physical. Picking up this cue, is there value in looking directly to the discipline of acting to find more ways to heighten our interpretive skills, our empathic connection, and our conceptual grasp of the process that unfolds in our work?

Mimesis as Method

In 1958 in her song "Showtime," the great blues and pop singer Dinah Washington told us that "the world is a showplace, and we all play our part" with the conviction and authenticity that made each of her performances indelibly true. In so doing, she repeated a metaphor that stretches back to the Renaissance, when Shakespeare told us in *As You Like It* (2.7), that "all the world's a stage" and that has become a defining theme of our postmodern age. There is something arresting about Dinah's commanding assertion, which came at a time when modernity still maintained its essentializing hold on most disciplines, notably psychoanalysis. She went on: "Well you want to be an actor, but you don't know how to act. . . . [No one tells me what to do in my show,] because in my show, Dinah's got the starring role!" In other words, if you want to play with me, you play by my rules. But how are we to understand the rules? How do we learn how to act? Well, yes, there are greater and lesser degrees of successful awareness of social cues, sensitivity to the affective states of others, empathic capacities. But, emphasizing and isolating for the moment the mimetic component of interpersonal experience, might there be a way to schematize, to practice the ability to learn one's part?

Perhaps inspired by Freud's various romantic descriptions of himself as a conquistador or an archaeologist, analysts have often given free rein to their wishes in constructing evocative professional identities. Spence (1987) posits a paradigm rooted in a legal metaphor. Others point out that the analyst is like a detective, rather more like Sherlock Holmes than Sam Spade one imagines. Recently analysts have been under siege by those who assert that because we cannot unequivocally construct ourselves as empirical scientists, we are practicing a fraudulent and charismatic kind of hokum (Grünbaum, 1984; Crews et al., 1998). But consider what we do when we analyze. At various times we perform tasks associated with all of these roles, and more. As infant researchers, some psychoanalysts are empirical scientists, and the insights they gather inform clinical work. Like detectives, we do try to understand a mystery; we collect evidence. Sometimes we even prosecute a case, though the analysand is probably not the defendant. Often we are cast in roles that we feel do not suit us, roles we become aware of only after the drama is underway.

When I assert that each of the three genres of my colleagues' stories is crucial to understanding the experience of the HIV-positive psychoanalyst, I am describing the importance of the analyst's versatility, another way of thinking about role responsiveness. As an analyst, one way to gain access to the experience of these stories is by imaginatively playing these widely ranging roles: Tamino or Florizel, Didi or Winnie, Frankenstein's creation, or Count Dracula. What kind of clinical and theoretical traction is generated if we embrace this infinitely capacious model of actor for the psychoanalyst?

The "Actor" metaphor appears in psychoanalytic literature often, to describe a variety of phenomena. Many analysts write about the analytic drama. Dimen (1998) refers to the body as "so much an actor, [that it] interrupts speech with a language of its own" (p. 66), a mimetic language. Grotstein (1994), arguing against disclosure in the treatment situation, asserts that

> from the standpoint of psychodrama, the application of the rule of abstinence follows the rules of dramaturgy—actors in any drama must totally abstain from being their conventional, known selves so that they can place themselves within the assigned roles of the characters they are portraying. Similarly, analysts must ascetically suspend their normal character behavior and must not share intimacies about their personal lives or opinions in general. Thus they behave in a disciplined role. Patients likewise play a role. Their freely associating selves are quite unlike themselves outside of the analytic setting. The very play-acting of these roles, based primarily on the abstinence of each "actor," is necessary, even mandatory, for the patient's therapeutic regression to take place and for the improvisational theatre of analysis to unfold [p. 605].

Grotstein is arguing from a one-person psychology point of view, in support of a classical technical stance. He stipulates that the therapeutic regression can take place only within an abstinent atmosphere. This is, I believe, a debatable point. It has been my experience that transference–countertransference manifestations beneficial to treatments have occurred within the context of the relatively nonabstinent atmosphere of my disclosures. Kent and Jasper are only two such examples. Further, his use of the metaphor of the actor overlooks some important aspects of the actual training processes that are available to contemporary actors. It is one rigorous method of acting training that I believe holds potentially innovative value for the analytic situation.

Like any sophisticated discipline, method acting is multifaceted. Stanislavsky's method (1989) has been interpreted by several American teachers. Two of the most prominent interpretations are from Sanford Meisner, who founded the Neighborhood Playhouse, and Lee Strasberg, who founded the Actors' Studio. Their versions of Stanislavsky's teachings are quite different, as I learned through my own training as an actor in classes taught from each point of view. Strasberg's exercises tend to focus on the actor in isolation, enabling greater access to personal memory and feeling, whereas Meisner's approach involves partnering with another. Like the divergence in psychoanalytic theories between the isolated mind of classical drive theory and the two-person model of contemporary relational schools of thought, the two versions of training for an actor are based in different theories of the art of representing the human. For Meisner, it was the moment-to-moment quality of a relationship that was the most fundamental element of the actor's art. For Strasberg, it was refining the actor's instrument (use of self) in isolation that was the first step. For Meisner, two bodies in space is the basic unit commanding our attention; for Strasberg, the actor begins with solo practice.

On the first day of the Meisner technique class that I took, our teacher told us that we needed to write down only one thing: that acting is behaving truthfully in imaginary circumstances and that the key to this craft is the reality of doing (Kareman, personal communication). *Doing* is the point. One cannot behave truthfully before another without doing.

Meisner's technique is based on what is commonly called the repeat exercise. In its most rudimentary form, partners stand opposite each other in silence until the one designated to begin feels prompted to make an observation about his partner. In the beginning, this may be something very simple, such as, "You are wearing a blue shirt." The partner repeats these words without consciously altering them in any way. The other then repeats the same words, as if automatically, in turn. And again, back and forth, many times. The repetition continues until transformations of the words occur spontaneously, without either partner's conscious manipulation. With time and practice, the partners' initial observations of each other will inevitably begin to include emotional states and intentions, but not because either partner sets out intentionally to do so. One of the important effects of the exercise is the growing ability to direct one's concentration onto the other so as to permit the emergence of the actor's emotional life without an inhibiting experience of self-consciousness.

The emotional life of the pair has a life of its own, which gradually becomes more prominent, inflecting each repetition, even as it changes with each repetition. The life of the pair can be thought of as a dialectic: one mind's idiomatic expression in response to the other, and the two minds coming to be in that particular way together. And neither is the life of the exercise reducible to either the two or the one; it is always already both.

What is it that happens in that first moment of the repeat exercise? In a way, the opening statement is something that occurs to all of us constantly. Some aspect of ourselves is noticed and remarked upon by another. This can be a benign event, or it can carry an affective charge. That moment when my doctor helpfully told me that as an HIV-positive person I was now a member of a community larger than many small cities, and the first comment to a naïve gay youth suggesting that he is "faggy," are both instances of this phenomenon. Although my doctor certainly did not intend it, my experience of that remark was one of separation, ejection, and isolation. For the young person who does not conform to gender roles, being called "faggy" can be devastating. An identity comes into being in these instances and is imposed on the subject of the remark. In Meisner's repeat exercise, the element of power, the traumatic aspect, is not the leading edge of the moment. But we can observe that an attribution is made that provokes either a revision of one's perception of oneself or an energetic rejection of the attribution. Either way, the subject is constituted for that moment through and by the other's declaration.

In the acting studio, the first partner might say, "You are wearing a blue shirt." This "you," the one wearing the blue shirt, is created in a particular relation to this other. "It is by this [blue shirt] that I know you as you, and that you will be known," the first actor is saying. This "you" then takes on the appellation: "I am wearing a blue shirt." "Yes," this new subject says, "I am this 'you' you have identified. So?" The originating other repeats his initial statement, and with the repetition there will be difference, an inflection that expresses something specific to that speaker, often of affective engagement. The reiteration of the original subjectivating statement by the subjectivating other opens the moment to a subjectivity of this first partner as well, a subjectivity indicated by another new inflection, of the difference of the repetition. And again the second partner repeats, again with a difference, another difference, and another elaboration of experience that is not premeditated, but is spontaneous, is excess, is beyond the words that are repeated by each of these newly constituted and reconstituting subjects.

The repeat exercise, when it is played by partners who have practiced sufficiently, ushers its players into pure process. Engaging in the exercise with an experienced partner is exhilarating, a surrendering to flux, constantly shifting, like riding an invisible wave. Working on it myself, I realized that Meisner's insight was that it is when the players most forget themselves that they are most alive, and he developed a systematic training in the practice of forgetting oneself. In this process of repetition, the quality of play relieves the subject of the anxiety of authenticity. The originating moment is not valued in itself as containing substance, but as setting off a series of relational experiences. A search for the meaning of a moment of origin, with an essential insight we must grasp, is revealed to be less important than that which we train our attention on so as to permit us to have a relationship.

The crucial dynamic of play reminds us that Winnicott (1969) devised what may be thought of as a different version of the repeat exercise, which he called "the squiggle game." Winnicott tells us that "in this squiggle game I make some kind of an impulsive line-drawing and invite the child whom I am interviewing to turn it into something, and then he makes a squiggle for me to turn into something in my turn" (p. 16). What Winnicott could observe was the child's capacity to play robustly, using another's gesture to create one of his or her own. That freedom to appropriate, in the context of play, is cultivated in the acting exercise.

The infant–caregiver research of Beebe (2002) is another psychoanalytic point of correspondence for the repeat exercise of the acting studio. In the videotaped vignettes of babies and their mothers from her studies, we witness a vast range of mothers' responses to their infants. Sometimes these moments are excruciating, as some mothers' anxieties mount when confronted with their infants' distress. These vignettes may be thought of as examples of failing to mirror, or an inability to repeat. Also recorded are Beebe's inspired matching of infant's facial expressions, breath and vocal rhythms. In these sequences we witness a process in which the previously distressed infants are calmed and engaged. What we see Beebe doing is mirroring an infant's physical and vocal expressions, repeating with a difference. As she does so, the infant responds with another version, another repetition. The pair engage in a nuanced conversation of facial and vocal inflections. It is tempting to think of Beebe's work, which involves a minutely detailed analysis of the mimetic relationship between infant and caregiver, as a primary instance of Meisner's repeat exercise.

This parallel has particular salience for those contemporary models of analytic process that emphasize the analyst's provision of holding and mirroring. Recent theorizing (e.g., Aron, 1996) on the value and use of the subjectivity of the analyst posits a generative dialectic relationship between these functions of mirroring and holding, and the introduction of the analyst's subjectivity. The Meisner method's repeat exercise is useful as a schematic for an intersubjective model. The analyst's act of placing his attention on the patient corresponds to the starting partner's neutral statement that begins the repeat exercise. Thinking of each exchange that follows this opening move—verbal or silent—as moments in which the subjectivities of each partner are always emerging spontaneously, alters our traditional conceptions of abstinence, anonymity, and disclosure. If we rethink our technique in terms of this ongoing emergence, an enactment or a brief moment of misattunement can become known less as a deviation or fault and more as an inevitable part of an unfolding process.

REPETITION AS A TRAUMATIC INSCRIPTION[1]

The repeat exercise also provides a method to isolate and observe what happens in the intersubjective space between people in moments when a quality, or an identity, is imposed on another, and whether and how that imposition is accommodated. Learning of one's HIV seropositivity has the impact of a traumatic inscription, often doubly traumatic when it is consistent with, and pursuant to, the management of a spoiled identity (Goffman, 1963), itself a traumatic inscription prior to HIV. Each inscription is another repetition. For HIV-positive gay men, for example, each descriptive term assigned to them has a narrative history, constructed in the myriad ways through which our culture is accumulated. With each new inscription, each repetition, our personal history is overwritten, elaborated. In the most traumatic of situations, the newly assigned identity can overwhelm any other narratives of identity. The subject is lost in toxic repetitions. An experience of being "written" in this way can have the impact of destroying what once appeared to be indestructible: that which is true about the self.

The registers of the intrapsychic and the interpersonal, or the private and social senses of identity, are mutually constitutive, and those marked by stigma are often subjects who may have been required to withstand repeated traumatic inscriptions. The social meanings of identity necessarily involve the social categories created by political forces, and these categories of identity have intrapsychic ramifications. Shifting to descriptions of the inauguration of the social subject as elaborated by Foucault (1980), formulated there as a process of *assujetissement* or subjectivation, and by Althusser (1971), as interpellation, we encounter variations on the theme of

---

[1] I am indebted to my friend and colleague Christopher B. Eldredge for our ongoing conversations on this idea.

traumatic inscription, the assignment of identity and the enforced accommodation of that assignment. Both describe the subject's coming into being, in greater and lesser ways into a deformed or defaced being, through the effects of power, often political power. The coming into being of a subject, in these paradigms, is not limited to marginal social identities but is common to us all. The effects of power are endlessly recirculated, repeated, as residual effects of the establishment of the norm.

Butler (1997), whose work has detailed the effects of power with regard to how gender and sexual roles are created and enforced, is acutely aware of the lethality of this process with regard to AIDS. She asks:

Can we read the workings of social power precisely in the delimitation of the field of such objects, objects marked for death? And is this part of the irreality, the melancholic aggression and the desire to vanquish, that characterizes the public response to the death of many of those considered "socially dead," who die from AIDS? Gay people, prostitutes, drug users, among others? If they are dying or already dead, let us vanquish them again. And can the sense of "triumph" be won precisely through a practice of social differentiation in which one achieves and maintains "social existence" only by the production and maintenance of those socially dead? [p. 27]

As both Foucault and Althusser depict the coming into being of the social subject, there is no question as to the subject's choice, because the very conditions of coming into being are determined by that power. Butler (1997) argues:

Bound to seek recognition of its own existence in categories, terms, and names that are not of its own making, the subject seeks the sign of its own existence outside itself, in a discourse that is at once dominant and indifferent. Social categories signify subordination and existence at once. In other words, within subjection the price of existence is subordination. Precisely at the moment in which choice is impossible, the subject pursues subordination as the promise of existence [p. 20].

I've reached for these descriptions of the ways that power and subordination are central to identity formation in both the sociopolitical register and the psychic, because a particularly disturbing kind of repetition has come to my attention in my work with Kent, when he told me, with some trepidation, about the sex he'd been having with a new romantic partner.

Articles reporting that some gay men engage in "barebacking" (having anal intercourse without condoms) have been appearing for some time, but this was the first occasion I'd had to respond to this question in my clinical work. Often these sexual partners are both HIV positive and can justify their practice on that basis. Others, HIV-negative gay men who call themselves "bug-chasers," are reported to seek out HIV-positive men, often via the internet, in order to have the virus passed on to them (Scarce, 1999). Cheuvront (2002) argues that if we can understand that such "risk-taking is not simply a function of individual character traits, but emerges in interpersonal contexts, then [we] are in the position to understand how, for example, risk-taking behavior can function as a solution to extinguish fear or anxiety, or how risk-taking behavior can ward off feelings of shame and humiliation, or how self-care can be suspended in the pursuit of desire" (p. 11). I would add that explanations of a kind of behavior that is extremely reckless require that we take into account not only psychoanalytic insights, but also the sociopolitical context in which the interpersonal world functions. Specifically, behavior that is self-destructive and that puts another person at risk of infection is one of a variety of repetitions related to the experience of a traumatically inscribed identity.

In the year after Kent recovered his dream of being buried alive next to his dead father, he experienced a period of expanded creativity and increased energy, expressed through his reconnection with his pleasure in drawing and painting. Yet he remained extremely unhappy and frustrated over his difficulties in finding appropriate men for romantic relationships. This reached a climax shortly before my summer vacation. With antidepressant medication, his mood stabilized and improved. When I returned from vacation, Kent reported that he'd begun a regular exercise program, which seemed to increase his sense of physical well-being. This contributed to a more robust sense of his emotional experience as well. He said that he felt more energetic. He began lifting weights for the first time and reported great satisfaction at noticing changes in his body, including a perceptible change in the "buffalo hump" that had long been an effect of the lipodystrophy brought on by his protease inhibitor. Whether this was due to a reduction of fat in his body or to better posture, he could not be sure, but he was very happy with his feeling that he was more attractive.

He also used various internet web sites to find ways to meet other men. He'd decided that risking rejection by HIV-negative men was too painful, so in his postings he clearly identified himself as HIV positive, interested in meeting other HIV-positive men. In the weeks immediately following my return from vacation, he described chatting with a few men he'd contacted this way, and then their first and second dates. Kent commented on the remarkable change in his social life, that after a long time during which he had not met anyone, he was dating several men.

Eventually, Kent told me he was seeing one man in particular, and that they had anal sex without a condom. His friend had told him that he didn't mind if Kent used a condom, but that he "was fine" if Kent did not. As Kent described these events, it appeared that he had left this decision to his new friend, not taking an active part in the decision himself. I asked about this aspect of the situation, and Kent confirmed that he thought that if it was all right with his friend, it was all right with him. He first told me this in a halting, shame-ridden way, and he clearly said he'd expected me to disapprove. In fact, I remained silent because I was struggling with how I might respond to what he'd told me. My own position has long been that, in light of all that we do not know, I cannot live with the possibility of putting anyone at risk through direct contact with my own semen or blood, whether or not the other is HIV positive. Yet I also am aware that for many, this stance places such frustrating limits on sexual behavior that it is sometimes impossible to maintain, and that many HIV-positive men engage in what is considered to be potentially risky sexual behavior together. For Kent, the leading edge of this problem was that making choices about his behavior could so easily become obscured by an active expression of desire by another.

Kent interpreted my silence as disapproval. I responded by asking if it was possible for us to consider, together, the various meanings that might be expressed through sexual behavior that we know poses at least a potential risk of reinfection to his partner. I was blunt: "What might fucking your friend without a condom mean?"

Kent was able to consider various meanings. He said first that it felt wonderful to experience again the freedom of sex as it had been before HIV/AIDS. I asked if it made any sense to connect themes that we had come to understand in our work with what he had just told me—themes about his despair and anger over not having felt taken care of and protected by me, particularly because his concern about my reaction to his having bareback sex related to the process through which he decided how to treat his new friend.

Kent was silent for a moment, thoughtful, and responded by asking if I meant that he might be expressing angry feelings by not using a condom. I asked him to say more about this idea. "Well, since B [his friend] is positive, maybe I see him as carrying the virus—as the virus—maybe, and so I am expressing my anger toward the virus by putting him at risk . . . But we really don't know how great that risk is."

"Yes, that is so," I said, "But can you say more about how he is the virus, somehow?"

"Oh, I don't know, really. . . . I was just thinking about my family, what we've talked about in the past, all the people, really, who disapprove of me—of gayness."

"Can you say more?"

"Maybe it's that because he is like me—he is positive—that this is a way of expressing anger at myself? That is so awful—here I've finally met someone who enjoys my company, who—we can have great sex together, and there's . . . this . . . this . . . I don't know. I don't like to think about it. Because I've finally found something that is enjoyable, even though B and I don't have all that much in common. But we do have a good time together."

If we can consider the impositions of identity that Kent refers to here as steps in the repetition of traumatic inscription, we can trace the struggle Kent is undergoing as he tries to narrate a new sense of himself as attractive, active, desirable. He has done a great deal of work on confronting the ways he has internalized, and repeats, his family's (and our culture's) homophobia. In a striking way, HIV has a sort of universally adhesive quality, and in Kent's case has taken over for internalized homophobia as a container for dissociated contents. Kent turned his attention to making certain reasonable changes in his appearance and vitality. In response, men he has been interested in have found him attractive. In turn, Kent's sense of being more attractive grows, along with a greater ease in asserting his wishes and interests, a repetition with a difference. But when it came to the matter of actually negotiating sexual contact with a partner, a subject saturated with meaning relating to HIV, what seemed to be repeated was a passive acceptance of the passive neglect of his partner. In an important way, passive neglect is an apt description of Kent's passive, depressed parents: a mother who in many ways enabled her husband to go on not working, even as he brought sexual partners home during the daytime when she was working two jobs. A dissociative mode of relating is a return to a familiar style. Repeating this style of relating may be the method for an expression of the dissociated murderous aggression that Kent has always needed to ward off. As we continue our work, we must keep track of the dissociated aspects of his story that are displaced into B, who, as an HIV-positive person, so readily takes on and repeats aspects of Kent's badness and vulnerability.

Within Kent's relationship to me, I often feel that I am drafted into the role of remaining unimpressed with, even disapproving of, the ways he finds pleasure. But here was a particularly difficult crisis point for me, one in which I ended up declaring my own ethical decisions. My silence was the first of a different kind of repetition: that of a relational moment in this episode. Remnants of an early traumatic inscription came to life as we repeated them, even as they have been kept alive by their repetition in the social norms throughout Kent's life. As we continued, I was aware of the necessity to leave room for an acknowledgment of the range of meanings that barebacking has for both of us, including the pleasurable, reality-denying aspects. But I found that the way I managed to do this included a frank description of my own position: a disclosure of how important it is for me to live with an ethical way of treating other people. It was another event that felt as though I were departing from standard technique. By disclosing my beliefs about appropriate sexual behavior, I established my presence more definitively. In order to bring into our relationship the problem of societal norms, perhaps I have to enact them (repeat them) myself through a clear description of my relationship to them. So I told him my position: that I could not live with the possibility that contact with my body fluids would endanger any sex partner. But through my enactment, I became aware that I was attempting a reinscription of a caring, responsible way of treating another, an alternative to the narrative that Kent repeats in which he is the neglected, abused victim. The inscription dynamic encompasses a vast range of ways to repeat.

Taking what happens in the social surround seriously, we can understand the enormous strain involved when existence is assured if the subject embraces as an identity a categorical norm that brings him or her into intelligibility by enacting the opposite of that norm. This episode centering on the question of bareback sex entails repetitions of moments inflected by Kent's experience with those on whom he'd depended as a child, which in turn had been repeated throughout Kent's widening circle of relationships and, of course, with me. When I repeat with a difference an exchange that includes the necessity for a conscious thinking through of how one treats others, I am both an old partner in repetitions, and a new one.

The task of the psychoanalytic situation is often described as helping the patient to find an authentic experience of the self, through this kind of encounter with new relational experiences. But how do we understand the sense of identity that comes into play through the accumulation of traumatic inscriptions, such as is suggested by Kent's history and style of relating, as authentic? Can we work our way out of this kind of traumatic inscription when our culture, including the culture of psychoanalysis, remains preoccupied with ideals of a substantial authenticity of identity?

THE PLATONIC IDEAL THAT HAUNTS IDEAS OF IDENTITY

Despite the descriptions of psychoanalytic concepts, such as Freud's tripartite model of the mind (id, ego, and superego as a dynamic system) or Kohut's invocation of mirroring, idealizing, and twinship selfobject needs as functions, there is a tendency for our understanding and use of these concepts to slide into reified forms. Drives seem to emanate from a place. A mirroring selfobject becomes the person performing that function rather than the mirroring action. It seems to be helpful to think of psychic systems and relationships as if they occupy space and have substance. Although it is often useful to gain therapeutic traction to use images of characters to talk about psychic events, there is the risk that this strategy can translate what are relational actions into substantial traits. What we are doing, usually for important and understandable reasons, becomes simply how we are, what we are made of. This translation from dynamics to substance lends a quality of immutability to our conceptions of identities, too.

Of course, we do have bodies, and so we conceive of ourselves in physical terms. But the difficulty thinking of ourselves as bodies and minds in action is partly a culturally determined phenomenon. To understand this further, I want to consider the manner in which Platonism, with its commitment to ideal forms transcending the vagaries of everyday existence, infiltrated psychoanalytic theory during the early decades of the last century. The ideal analyst emerged in various ways: the ways our literature defined standard technique, specifically the values of neutrality and anonymity, relying on metaphors like that of the surgeon and the mirror. The ways that the analyst's vulnerability is set aside, dissociated, in our discourse implies a similar ideal guiding our identifications as analysts. This way we have of reaching after an ideal that resides out there somewhere repeats the action of Platonic knowing through contact with an ideal form.

Specifically it is Plato's (n.d.) theory of ideas (which assumes that every object and idea can be judged against its original, ideal form) that some argue is not descriptive, but prescriptive, and that has left an abiding influence on the problem of how we locate an authentic ground for our being. Heidegger mounted a detailed critique of the effects of what he diagnosed as the dominance of Platonic ideality. He asserted that the "ontotheology," a "religion of being" that began with Plato, rests in a way of thinking that is "either overtly or covertly metaphysical. 'What characterizes metaphysical thinking . . . is the fact that [it] departs from what is present and thus represents it in terms of its ground as something grounded'" (cited in Taylor, 1987, p. xxvi). It is as if Heidegger complains that under the influence of Plato, philosophers—for all their questions about the world—have forgotten that the world, and human beings performing actions within it, actually exists.

Understanding how the model of Plato's ideality of form is still influential helps us to notice how the repetition of a norm is transposed into a fiction of genuine essence. We enact this project by building up a narrative of continuing identity, relying on analogy and accumulating an expanding body of historical figures on which to found a substantial essence. By analogy, I point to the link between a sense of gay identity, and what became the movement to support those with HIV/AIDS, and the eventual development of something called an HIV-positive identity. Faced with a fight for our lives, we turned to the social and political structures that had also provided an armature for an identity that had enabled gay people to come into existence as social subjects that matter. Of course, the gay movement had itself relied, in important ways, on the models of the civil rights and feminist movements, and, as Bersani (1988) reminds us, this is a relationship that continues to be elaborated. What I seek to emphasize here is the way that social and political dimensions of identity play a crucial constitutive role in the formation of identities experienced as private and intrapsychic. These sources of contemporary identity are derived from liberatory, ethical, political and social motives, and these motives are obscured by the search for a gay identity grounded in a Platonic ideality. Recently, this ideal form has been tailored to mimic a North American middle-class norm, and is accomplished through appeals to a variety of discourses.

For example, one way an ideal form for gay identity has been constructed is through a process that includes the appropriation of historical figures to whom the contemporary notion of a gay person would have been unintelligible. Claiming Elizabethan playwright Christopher Marlowe, for example, as a gay forebear, depends on a very selective understanding of the world in which he lived. Although our world may share a number of features with Marlowe's, particularly the establishment of a discrete group through the suppression of specific sexual acts (Foucault, 1978), differences between these worlds tend to be minimized in what becomes built up, through repetition, into a norm. (See Bray, 1982, on Renaissance England differing with Foucault on the existence of an identifiable group based on erotic preference.) And though it may be true that there are more commonalities than differences between the experience of gay men today and men who had sex with men in 1570, the building up of historical citations of gay identity begins to resemble a process of subjectivation in retrospect. It is a repetition of the use of power to establish a claim of legitimacy, in response to our own traumatic inscription.

The recent claims for a physiological and biological cause for homosexual behavior (Hamer and Copeland, 1994) is another example of an appeal to Platonic ideality. One way we have of coping with alienation from a grounded sense of being is the building up of substantial constituents of identity that express an essence we'd prefer to think of as biologically derived. A biologically determined identity somehow seems more true, more defensible. In our contemporary scientific world, biology functions as a form of the ideal.

The different versions of identities that I have explored throughout this project—the personal, the social, the sexual, the political— are determined, to a greater or lesser degree, by comparison with an ideal form of each. If we could establish a link with the ideal, find an essence, we'd be relieved of some of the trauma of being written by another. But even the prideful search for an authentic identity can turn into a search for an elusive ideal that keeps escaping, like an errant ball of mercury. One patient came to treatment with an awful feeling that he wasn't able to be "gay enough." The concept of identity itself amounted, for him, to an imposition of an ideal form, which in turn left him obsessed with an ideal that remains forever beyond his grasp.

Lorde (1982) depicted the progress of this obsessive search for an authenticity of identity, and the acknowledgment that difference *is* the very ground for our experience:

> Being women together was not enough. We were different. Being gay-girls together was not enough. We were different. Being Black together was not enough. We were different. Being Black women together was not enough. We were different. Being Black dykes together was not enough. We were different. . . . It was a while before we came to realize that our place was the very house of difference rather than the security of any one particular difference [p. 226].

How do we come to realize that we cannot *find* this "house of difference" because we've always lived there? Is psychoanalysis, practiced in a register of doing rather than being, one means of coming to this awakening? Waking to the notion that we are already living in a house of difference, I hasten to add, does not require an experience of any particular condition. But often a stigmatized condition is the impetus for what can feel like a rude awakening.

REPETITION AND IDENTITY

In a sense, method acting training is Heideggerian in that it seeks to dismantle Platonic ideality, moving away from stock figures in drama toward the specificity of particular individuals. The method was developed in response to styles of acting that depended on an immediate recognition of stereotypes, of identities that were worn like signs. Affects, too, were indicated by behavioral signs: emotion was either indicated in crude and regimented ways, as in the 19th-century Del Sarte charts of rhetorical acting that illustrated poses and expressions suitable for the emotion to be conveyed, or garishly displayed with little sense of any connection with a believable narrative, as in the wild emoting of early melodrama. The famous exceptions, known to us now only in contemporary descriptions and rare film clips of actors such as Duse, Bernhardt, and Kean, may be those that prove this rule about premethod acting styles. We must also rely on the complaints made by Stanislavsky (1989).

As I learned in classes that taught Meisner's technique, the craft of portraying characters rests on this important insight: whatever it is that makes the individual specific is beyond our grasp. The individual's idiomatic selfhood is most apparent when the individual is least conscious of being or presenting it, and emerges in relation to another. The method seeks to account for the unconscious. But acting teachers know that it is only through a realistic doing that the unconscious is expressed as it inflects behavior.

Meisner's basic training tool, the repetition exercise, by focusing on actions that express, points up how lacking in substance an "identity" is. Meisner's emphasis on *doing* echoes Nietzsche's (1888) claim that "there is no 'being' behind doing, effecting, becoming; 'the doer' is merely a fiction added to the deed—the deed is everything" (p. 45). The notion of identity as a category is revealed to be inert and empty without a doing.

The rule-bound and fluidly changeable playacting of children shows us the tension this emptiness causes, as well as our spontaneous capacity to fill categories of identity. For if identity is a necessary fiction, what keeps the fiction going if not the social dimension? The rules that mark identity allow for fluid movement among identities. For children, a daddy does certain things because he is the daddy, and so with mommies, policemen, aliens, and dinosaurs. Our abhorrence of the vacuum of identity is ceaselessly elaborated. Analysts, of course, make use of our tendency to fill this vacuum by seeking to remain relatively free of markers of subjective identity.

This is a complicated project. That very seeking for a relatively anonymous presentation is a form of doing, a means of communicating. Just what is communicated, or understood by the patient, is often the topic of early interpretations. Analysands all have their own ways of responding to a relatively anonymous analyst, and for many analysts, the ways their patients respond is an important source of data. But regardless of theoretical allegiance, the subjectivity of any analyst is constantly leaking out. The manner in which one dresses or decorates one's office is either an expression of subjectivity or an attempt to minimize that expression (Goldstein, 1994, 1997). Thus, the analyst is performing—doing—consciously or not, a characterization of himself or herself as analyst for presentation to the patient. Schafer (1983) has described a second version of that function as the analyst: as analysts, one is a better person than in private life. The analyst/actor's preparation involves these components: readying oneself to be used by the analysand and creating a version of oneself through the self-conscious doing of presentation. It is the latter that was, for a time, subsumed by the analytic ideal of the blank slate, and it is the background against which contemporary analysts are theorizing alternatives.

The repeat exercise is an alternative that may permit the analyst's preparation to become more conscious and explicit. Preparation using the repeat exercise would provide analysts with an experience of improvising with another person. Often this improvisation consists of matching the affective state of the partner. In the work of such researchers as Beebe and her colleagues (Beebe and Lachmann, 2002), affective matching has been shown to be crucial to infant–caregiver interaction. The repeat exercise allows analysts to develop skills in affective matching. This is perhaps the strongest link between acting training and the clinical situation conceived in an intersubjective mode.

The exercise is also helpful in reducing a beginning analyst's self-consciousness. I recall my own experience with the exercise prior to analytic training, when I found it to be helpful in training my concentration away from myself, directing it onto my partner in order to attend more closely to that person's communications and affective state. The exercise helps with losing concentration on self in order to fall into the jointly created experience between the two partners.

Shifting from practice to theory, the repeat exercise also functions as a highly overdetermined metaphor. It is a description of the viruslike communicability and infinite variation of dissociated and disowned psychic experience. Functioning as an analytic tool, the concept of repetition helped me to think through, in a detailed way, a process I've referred to as traumatic inscription. In this context, I could theorize how traumatic inscription (being written) works in the formation of identity as well as its implication in such difficult clinical issues as that described in the example of Kent and bareback sex.

Finally, there is a personal dynamic at work in the concept of the repetition exercise that makes this theatrical metaphor compelling to me. Developing this metaphor to theorize aspects of my experience as an analyst serves to reestablish a connection with a past version of myself, a lifelong fascination and involvement with the theatre that has been subordinated to my psychoanalytic work. I've come to understand that this theme springing back to life enacts its own promise of transformation: it imparts a sense of both ongoing continuity and constant change, of new timbers replacing old, evoking a sense of aliveness and creativity.

The reestablishment of this link with my past experience vitalizes the process of integrating psychoanalytic technique and theory into the construction of an identity conceived as a doing. Another repetition: an enactment of what I'm trying to describe, that recovering aspects of a former relationship to creativity and aliveness makes me both more nearly the same and more different. And to recover from the traumatic inscription of HIV seropositivity, I dismantle an identity in order to articulate an unfolding relationship in action. As Barthes (1977) suggests, the gradual replacement of the timbers of the Argo describes the empowering potential effects of substitution and nomination. This also works as a schematic of the shimmer of dialectic tension between the register of ideal, genuine forms and the fluidity of relational activity.

I wish to push the metaphor further. I propose that the repetition exercise points the way to make the doing of psychoanalysis freer of the substantive ideal of being a psychoanalyst, and that this in turn enables a rethinking of the question of disclosure.

COMING OUT AND THE PSYCHOANALYST: DISCLOSURE AS REPETITION

Disclosure is a coming out of sorts. Disclosure in a psychoanalytic setting, such as my disclosures of HIV status, repeats the daily coming out of lesbian, gay, bisexual, and transgendered people. In making this link between disclosure and coming out, I am conscious of drawing attention not only to the action of revealing private information, but also to the repetition and exploitation of a nodal point that is central to one valence of the dynamic meanings surrounding HIV/AIDS, and that is sex. I object to use of the phrase "coming out" in this way, even as I choose to use it in the interest of making myself understood. By linking disclosure and coming out, I am also implying the associative linkage of HIV/AIDS with gay male sex. And, of course, I have been doing this all along.

Although this association now inaccurately describes the majority of those who will become infected with HIV/AIDS in the time it takes to read this, HIV/AIDS has become fixed in general knowledge as linked to gay male sexuality. Although it is true that infection has become a normal, expected part of life for many gay men in urban settings, the persistent and apparently permanent notion that HIV/AIDS equals gay male sexuality is inaccurate in the developing world, where it is now predominantly a disease of women and children. In the winter of 1999, the baseball player John Rocker infamously repeated this linkage in his description of riding the subway through a part of New York City, where a "fag with AIDS" might be seated next to him. The more we repeat this linkage, the truer and more transparent it becomes, and the more we obscure what is accurate.

Coming out is a compelling metaphor for many possible secrets. It has entered popular usage as a designation for any disclosure that is anxiety ridden. However, as most homosexual men and women know it, coming out is not a discrete event, but an interpersonal decision that is negotiated—repeated—every day. In clinical situations, in my private life, in casual conversations, it is always already there (like my seropositivity), forcing a negotiation that begins in the privacy of my thoughts and usually becomes known to another. It is this aspect—this omnipresent, ongoing process of coming out—that I wish to emphasize.

I have observed that many patients describe their experience before coming out as something like this: There is a gap between each of them and the rest of the world. This gap comprises the way(s) in which they are not understood, or the way(s) it will be impossible to feel understood, by others. Perhaps they feel as if they will be understood after coming out. Perhaps that is precisely the problem: they will be understood too well and dismissed or worse. Or, once they are understood, they are understandable to themselves, and there is relief. A person may approach the edge of this gap, may feel on the verge of crossing over it to the other side, and then may identify a feeling of belonging there. That may be a good idea or a bad idea. Either way, there is a sense of finally being understood, of being identified and becoming identifiable. Either way, repetitions of a dreaded belief are confronted.

Is this series of anxious propositions applicable to the analyst who discloses? The traditional analyst, who has been invested in maintaining anonymity and in sustaining a tabula rasa on which to permit all of the patient's projections and fantasies to register and to be repeated in the controlled environment of the analysis would not think so. A coming out or a disclosure would result in disrupting the repetitions in the transference. Being understood in a new way through disclosures would diminish his or her effectiveness.

But this point of view emphasizes only continuity. An alternative approach to disclosing or coming out would include the value of novelty and change. If we regard a disclosure as the opening move in a series, a chain of relational events, we might expect not to be understood, but to see how misunderstood we may continue to be, an emphasis on the difference that always remains. Regarded in this way, any disclosure carries with it an implicit and paradoxical acknowledgment of both continuity and change. Continuity and change coexist, as in the moments of the repeat exercise in which the idioms of the partners generate changes with each repetition.

The analyst who is faced with the problem of helping a patient work through a traumatic inscription is often faced with a dilemma concerning the terrors of change and flexibility. Often the alternative to a traumatic inscription is an authenticity that seems to be inspired, to one degree or another, by a Platonic ideal that is impossible to attain. Like many men's difficult experience of gender role as they attempt to enact the masculine, such an ideal sets in motion an obsessive quest in which at least the continuity of strain resides

(Pleck, 1995). In this context, perhaps the analyst's disclosure presents an opportunity to undermine those narratives of identity that bring suffering. Psychoanalytic theories describe expressions of suffering in various ways. Symptoms can be associated with acute trauma or chronically ill-attuned parenting, as compromise formations attempting to resolve conflicts arising from repressed sexual fantasy, as character armor that evolved to manage a terrifying inner object world, or as a combination of these with socio-political dynamics of subjectivation. Often the experience of symptoms is experienced by patients as an identity, and can be thought of as a narrative that has been developed in an attempt to maintain ongoing safety, to make one understandable to oneself, and to survive in the world. To call this a narrative is in no way to suggest that it is inauthentic. Such a narrative, understood as a response to traumatic inscription, is developed out of dire necessity, and there is no sense of there being any other option available. Predictability and safety lie in the repetition of what has been inscribed.

But the unique privilege the psychoanalyst claims is to point out that the narrative that has evolved in response to traumatic inscription may not be the only option from this point on, particularly when we pay attention to what the narrative leaves out. If identity is a relational process of constant reinscription, of repetitions with a difference, then it may be possible to reorganize one's narrative to include the value of flexibility as well as continuity. What once was convincingly understood will be pointedly misunderstood, or rather reunderstood, in the service of undermining the sense that there is only one way of understanding oneself. I have found that in my work, coming out as HIV-positive is an opening move in this process of finding ways to help patients conceive new styles of narrative. My HIV seropositivity challenges not only my ideal form of the psychoanalyst, but my patients' as well. Repeating with a difference an imposed identity brings onto our stage the opportunity to consider our tendency to repeat what we have been required not to know.

The American relational school of analysis is particularly concerned with the question of authenticity. If one characteristic narrative style of an individual's experience is not the *only* possible narrative style, what can we regard as authentic? My experience of Meisner's repeat exercise showed me compellingly that convincing individuality is evoked through the repetition of an action. The exercise points out that authenticity is not something one can possess or contain; it is located not in a discrete substance of an identity, but in the elusive beyond intimated in the accumulation of repetitions. To what extent is it possible to know that we are known? At the very best, we can agree to a mutual, consensual negotiation of self and other (Pizer, 1998). That negotiation is one action we perform in a relationship, and it is through that action that our idiomatic particularity is expressed, whether we set out to do so or not. To regard what we come to understand through the process of negotiated repetitions as final, substantial, known once and for all, is to commit continual violence on the other, on the order of the traumatic inscription of identity.

So when a disclosure, a coming out, carries with it an awareness of the possibility, even the utility, of being misunderstood, because it is regarded as an opening move in a series of repetitions, it becomes an opportunity for a creative retranscription. To be sure, what is made known may be expanded but paradoxically the new information also opens a gap. We must come to grips with a new difference between self and other as well as between self and new self-experience. We encounter the limit of the known. A disclosure can lead to a moment of destabilization that provides for the analytic subject a chance to expand creative potential, a period of freedom to experience himself as responding with greater freedom and flexibility. Optimal moments of destabilization, carried in repetitions in which continuity and change coincide, are experiences like riding on a wave, like Barthes's (1977) realization that all of his timbers have been replaced, and like those wonderful and terrible moments when a difference makes itself known through a crack in the everyday: a dream, a slip of the tongue. The action of HIV, too, is an iteration and an elaboration in each of its accumulated repetitions of mutation.

As analysts, we find ways to work toward that experience of riding a crest of change with our patients, to glimpse together the possibility for revising a traumatic inscription so that it loses its substantive finality as the way things are. In clinical work practiced in a mode of doing rather than being, both analyst and analysand become more expert at forgetting themselves, gaining the confidence that the more we dare to surrender to the action of mutual repetitions, the more present we will be.

Afterword

Being HIV positive has challenged me to become aware of the shimmering dialectical tension of each moment of our lives, what Hoffmann (1998) refers to when he invokes the "dialectic of meaning and mortality" (p. 18). As with any loss, my HIV-positive status often acts like a spur, a goad that reminds me not to take anything for granted. This is one way that HIV seropositivity keeps pushing me out of any special category, rather than shutting me in a private club. And so, if there is a story to be found in the unpacking of the complicated meanings of my seropositivity, I hope that it contributes to an understanding of the psychoanalytic process generally, and that is is not read as limited to the specific condition of HIV seropositivity.

It was out of the specific condition of seropositivity that I confronted the problem of disclosure, but it quickly opened out into broader significance. I discovered that general recommendations on disclosures proved to be less helpful to me than the detailed stories of the disclosures of other analysts, a kind of story that has become available only relatively recently. These stories are often examples of clinicians who felt themselves pushed to a limit of one kind or another. Limit cases often tend to stretch the boundary around what we know, allowing us to encroach on what has yet to be understood. Each particular story depends on a subsequent story, a repetition with a difference, to further this expansion and accumulation of insight.

In his radical experiments with mutual analysis, Ferenczi (1933) presented us with the ultimate test case on disclosure. The goal of establishing mutuality was predicated on a fully equal exchange. Such equality proved to be unsustainable. But the value of finding ways to acknowledge the analyst's mutual involvement in the analytic process endures. In a sense, making a disclosure is expressive of this value, and so it is like an embrace. When we approach the question of disclosure as action, part of a chain of moments, our attention is directed to the process of meaning making. Doing so, our work becomes more complicated, but also, I believe, more useful. It has been my experience that the most transformative aspect of the disclosures I have made had to do with the unfolding process following that moment, and that the content of my disclosures was of secondary importance, used in the service of that process.

Similarly, identities that have been established for important strategic sociopolitical, as well as psychological, reasons and motives are not so reliably durable and discrete. When we look at an island on a map, we see a discrete entity. But of course, the edge of the island is really a beach, an ever-changing, permeable interpenetration of sand and water. Like the boundary of an island, identity is a dynamic process, a shifting, relational construction rather than a description of some psychic content. There is tremendous importance in understanding and confronting the strategic uses of the notion of identity. The intersection of social theory, politics, and psychoanalysis is a complicated location in which to attend to the prevailing processes at work. Identities live when they are dynamic, moving in relation to another. The question, "Who are you?" is far less effective in gathering information than, "What is it that you are you doing and how are you doing it?"

I do not wish to minimize the importance of the universal experience of selfhood (an experience that often includes a sense of durable contents), but to point out how selfhood is expressed and becomes knowable through participation in a process. It is a matter of striving for a dialectical sense of oneself that involves an imminent sense of being made up of certain contents that can only be experienced through a process of doing.

As Corbett (2001) puts it, the practice of psychoanalysis has the potential for embracing more life, an expansive inclusion of the margins, of continuity and change, countering the dubious comforts of the normal. When I first encountered Freud's work, it appealed to me because of the convincing way he undermined any such category as normal. The ongoing challenge for psychoanalysis is whether its embrace can include the awareness that we are always living in the house of difference. Approaching certain disclosures as expressive of this awareness is one way to acknowledge this. I believe psychoanalysis is particularly well suited to meet this challenge, becoming a voice of resistance to the tendency to reify processes into structures that have an enduring, true essence.

The history of HIV/AIDS shows that it is just one phenomenon that has become elaborated as a pretext for an identity politics that depends on a presumed genuine core residing in that identity. When identities are fixed and immutable, otherness tends to be experienced as alien. The split world of either–or has little room for the ordinary, the wonderfully human, in a clinical sense as well as in a broader perspective of the world in which we all live. We suffer from the lethal strategic stigmatization and exploitation of difference; we see all too often that it is a matter of life and death.

Appendix A

Sample Letter sent to Chairpersons of Professional Societies of Psychoanalytic Training Institutes

Dear Colleague,

I write to you today to describe a project with which I require assistance, in the hope that you may be able to provide it. I am seeking partners in research for a study on the analyst's experience of being HIV seropositive, and the influence that this condition may have on clinical work. I'm hoping to locate other HIV-positive analysts who would agree to one or two interviews of not longer than 90 minutes. The interviews would be structured only by the theme of whether and how being HIV positive has exerted an influence on the work. All participants will receive a transcript of the interview for their approval, and, of course, in any written communication based on the interviews, all identifying data will be thoroughly disguised, in conformity with APA standards.

It is my hope that you might pass along the word of my project to any analysts whom you might know who would be interested and willing to participate in the research. The phone number listed above is the best way to contact me.

I am mindful of the delicacy of such a request. The study will be conducted in such a way as to preserve the anonymity of all participants. In the service of maintaining anonymity in the process of locating potential research partners, I enclose a notice describing the research study for posting in an area where members of your society or clinic would be likely to see it. Any assistance you may be able to provide for this project is gratefully valued.

Appendix B

Sample Letter sent to members of GALA (Gay and Lesbian Analysts)

Dear Colleague,

I write to you today with a request, presuming on our common membership in GALA. I am in the process of designing a qualitative research project that seeks to inquire into the experience of the psychoanalyst who is HIV-positive. The focus will be on doing clinical work as an HIV-positive person and any potential effects that the condition of seropositivity may exert on the treatment relationship. In order to gather data for the study, I must locate analysts who are HIV positive. The subjects must have formal analytic training. The interviews will be no longer than 90 minutes in length and will be structured by the theme of the analyst's experience in clinical work. Participants will receive transcripts of the interviews for their approval. The project design will conform to APA standards for research. All interview material will be confidential. In the writeup of the research data, any identifying data will be thoroughly disguised.

As you might imagine, it has been a challenge to identify potential partners in research. It is my hope that, should you know of an analyst who is HIV positive who may be interested in participating in this study, you will alert them to the project. They may contact me at [phone number].

I appreciate any assistance you are able to provide.

APPENDIX C

SAMPLE FLYER MAILED FOR POSTING AT PSYCHOANALYTIC TRAINING INSTITUTES

Seeking Subjects for Research Project
on
the Analyst's Experience of Being
HIV Seropositive
in the practice of
Psychoanalysis and Psychoanalytic Psychotherapy

*   *   *   *

I am seeking Psychoanalysts and Psychoanalytic Psychotherapists who are HIV positive for a project that seeks to expand the understanding of the experience of the HIV-positive analyst, and any possible influences of the analyst's HIV seropositivity on clinical practice. Interviews of no longer than 90 minutes will be structured only by the theme of the Analyst's experiences in clinical work and whether and how the condition of being HIV positive has affected the work with patients. Participants will receive transcripts of interviews for approval. All interview material will be confidential, and any identifying data will be thoroughly disguised in the completed study.
Should you be interested in participating, please contact:
Gilbert W. Cole
[phone number]

REFERENCES

Abend, S. (1982), Serious illness in the analyst: Countertransference considerations. *J. Amer. Psychoanal. Assn.*, 30:365–379.

———— (1986), Countertransference, empathy, and the analytic ideal: The impact of life stresses on analytic capability. *Psychoanal. Quart.*, 55:536–575.

Aldington, R. & Ames, D. (1959), *The New Larousse Encyclopedia of Mythology* London: Hamlyn.

Alien (1979), Film. Hollywood, CA: 20th Century Fox.

Alien Resurrection (1997), Film. Hollywood, CA: 20th Century Fox.

Aliens (1986), Film. Hollywood, CA: 20th Century Fox.

Alien³ (1992), Film. Hollywood, CA: 20th Century Fox.

Althusser, L. (1971), Ideology and ideological state apparatuses (Notes toward an investigation). In *Lenin and Philosophy and Other Essays.* tr. B. Brewster. New York: Monthly Review Press.

American Psychological Association (1992), *Ethical Principles of Psychologists and Code of Conduct.* Washington, DC: American Psychological Assn.

Aristotle (n. d.). *Nichomachean Ethics.* tr. D.Ross. Oxford: Oxford University Press.

Arlow, J. (1990), The analytic attitude in the service of denial. In *Illness in the Analyst: Implications for Treatment,* ed. H. J. Schwartz & A. L. Silver. New York: International Universities Press, 1990, pp. 9–26.

Aron, L. (1996), *A Meeting of Minds.* Hillsdale, NJ: The Analytic Press.

Aronson, S. (1996), The bereavement process in children of parents with AIDS. *Psychoanalytic Study of the Child,* 51:422–435. New Haven CT: Yale University Press.

Bauknight, R. & Appelbaum, R. (1997), AIDS, death, and the analytic frame. *Free Associations,* 41(A):81–100.

Barthes, R. (1970), *S/Z.* New York: Hill & Wang.

———— (1977), *Barthes by Barthes.* New York: Hill & Wang.

Beckett, S. (1954), *Waiting for Godot.* New York: Grove Press.

———— (1961), *Happy Days.* New York: Grove Press.

Beebe, B. & Lachmann, F. (2002), *Infant Research and Adult Treatment: Co-constructing Interactions.* Hillsdale, NJ: The Analytic Press.

Benjamin, J. (1988), *The Bonds of Love: Psychoanalysis, Feminism, and the Problem of Domination.* New York: Pantheon.

———— (1995), *Like Subjects, Love Objects*. New Haven CT: Yale University Press.

Bersani, L. (1988), Is the rectum a grave? In: *AIDS: Cultural Analysis/Cultural Activism*, ed. D. Crimp. Cambridge, MA: MIT Press. pp. 197–222.

Blechner, M. J. (1993), Psychoanalysis and HIV disease. *Contemp. Psychoanal.*, 29:61–80.

———— (1997a), Psychological aspects of the AIDS epidemic: a fifteen-year perspective. *Contemp. Psychoanal.*, 33:89–107.

———— (ed.) (1997b), *Hope and Mortality: Psychodynamic Approaches to AIDS and HIV*. Hillsdale, NJ: The Analytic Press.

Bloom, H. (1965), Afterword. In *Frankenstein, or the Modern Prometheus* by M. Shelley. New York: Signet Classic.

Blos, P. (1967), The second individuation process of adolescence. In *The Psychology of Adolescence: Essential Readings*, ed. A. Esman. Madison CT: International Universities Press, 1975, pp. 165–176.

Bollas, C. (1987), *The Shadow of the Object*. New York: Columbia University Press.

Bowie, M. (1991), *Lacan*. Cambridge, MA: Harvard University Press.

Boyarin, D. (1997), *Unheroic Acts: The Rise of Heterosexuality and the Invention of the Jewish Man*. Berkeley: University of California Press.

Bram Stoker's Dracula (1992), Film. Hollywood, CA: Columbia Tri Star.

Bray, A. (1982), *Homosexuality in Renaissance England*. London: Gay Men's Press.

Breuer, J. & Freud, S. (1893–1895), *Studies in Hysteria. Standard Edition*, 2. London: Hogarth Press, 1955.

Bromberg, P. (1998), *Standing in the Spaces: Essays on Clinical Process, Trauma and Dissociation*. Hillsdale, NJ: The Analytic Press.

Brudnoy, D. (1997), *Life is Not a Rehearsal: A Memoir*. New York: Doubleday.

Butler, J. (1997), *The Psychic Life of Power: Theories of Subjection*. Stanford, CA: Stanford University Press.

Chermin, P. (1976), Illness in a therapist—Loss of omnipotence. *Arch. Gen. Psychiat.*, 33:1327–1328.

Cheuvront, J. P. (2002), High-risk sexual behavior in the treatment of HIV negative patients. *J. Gay & Lesbian Psychotherapy*, 3:7–25.

Clinical Social Work Federation (1997), Code of Ethics. Clinical Social Work Federation: Arlington, VA.

Cohen, J. & Abramowitz, S. (1990), AIDS attacks the self: A self-psychological exploration of the psychodynamic consequences of HIV. *The Realities of Transference: Progress in Self Psychology, Vol. 16*. Hillsdale NJ: The Analytic Press, pp. 157–172.

Corbett, K. (2001), More life: Centrality and marginality in human development. *Psychoanal. Dial.*, 11:313–336.

Craft, C. (1984), Kiss me with those red lips: Gender and inversion in *Dracula*. *Representations*, 8:109–110.

Crapanzano, V. (1992), *Hermes' Dilemma and Hamlet's Desire: On the Epistemology of Interpretation*. Cambridge, MA: Harvard University Press.

Crespi, L. (1995), Some thoughts on the role of mourning in the development of a positive lesbian identity. In *Disorienting Sexuality*. ed. T. Domenici & R. Lesser. New York: Routledge, 1995, pp. 19–32.

Crews, F., Blum, H. P., Cavell, M., Eagle, M., Crews, Freda (eds.) (1995), *The Memory Wars: Freud's Legacy in Dispute*. New York: New York Review Books.

Davies, J. (1994), Love in the afternoon. *Psychoanal. Dial.*, 4:503–508.

——— (2000), Descending the therapeutic slopes——Slippery, slipperier, slipperiest: Commentary on papers by Barbara Pizer and Glen O. Gabbard. *Psychoanal. Dial.*, 10:219–230.

Derrida, J. (1978), *Writing and Difference*, tr. Alan Bass. Chicago: University of Chicago Press.

Dewald, P. (1982), Serious illness in the analyst: Transference, countertransference and reality responses. *J. Amer. Psychoanal. Assn.*, 30:347–363.

Dimen, M. (1995), On "Our Nature": Prologomenon to a relational theory of sexuality. In *Disorienting Sexuality: Psychoanalytic Reappraisals of Sexual Identities*, ed. T. Domenici & R. Lesser. New York: Routledge, 1995, pp. 129–152.

——— (1998), Polyglot bodies: Thinking through the relational. In *Relational Perspectives on the Body*, ed. L. Aron & F. Anderson. Hillsdale, NJ: The Analytic Press, 1998, pp. 65–93.

Doty, M. (1996), *Heaven's Coast: A Memoir*. New York: Harper Collins.

Drescher, J. (1999), *Psychotherapy and the Gay Man*. Hillsdale, NJ: The Analytic Press.

Duberman, M. (1994), *Stonewall*. New York: Dutton.

Durban, J., Lazar, R., & Ofer, G. (1993), The cracked container, the containing crack: Chronic illness—its effect on the therapist and the therapeutic process. *Internat. J. Psycho-Anal.*, 74:705–713.

Eckstein, R. (1976), Psychoanalysis and education as allies in the acquisition of moral values and virtues in the service of peace. *Internat. Rev. Psycho-Anal.*, 3:399–408.

Edelson, M. (1984), *Hypothesis and Evidence in Psychoanalysis*. Chicago: University of Chicago Press.

Ehrenberg, D. (1995), Self-disclosure: Therapeutic tool or indulgence? Countertransference disclosure. *Contemp. Psychoanal.* 31:213–228.

Erikson, E. (1964), *Insight and Responsibility: Lectures on the Ethical Implications of Psychoanalytic Insight*. New York: Norton.

——— (1976), Psychoanalysis and ethics—Avowed and unavowed. *Internat. Rev. Psycho-Anal.*, 3:409–414.

Esslin, M. (1961), *The Theatre of the Absurd*. New York: Anchor Books.

Fast, I. (1998), *Selving: A Relational Theory of Self Organization*. Hillsdale, NJ: The Analytic Press.

Feinberg, D. (1995), *Queer and Loathing: Rants of an AIDS Clone*. New York: Penguin.

Ferenczi, S. (1932), *The Clinical Diary of Sandor Ferenczi*, ed. J. Dupont (tr. M. Baltin & N. Z. Jackson). Cambridge, MA: Harvard University Press, 1988.

——— (1933), Confusion of tongues between adults and children. In: *Final Contributions to the Problems and Methods of Psycho-analysis*. New York: Bruner/Mazel, 1980, pp. 156–166.

Foucault, M. (1973), *The Birth of the Clinic*. New York: Vintage.

———— (1978), *The History of Sexuality, Vol. I: An Introduction*. New York: Random House.

———— (1980), *Power/Knowledge: Selected Interviews and Other Writings*. New York: Pantheon.

Freud, S. (1900), *The Interpretation of Dreams. Standard Edition*, 4–5. London: Hogarth Press, 1955.

———— (1905a), *Three essays on sexuality. Standard Edition*, 7:123–246. London: Hogarth Press, 1955.

———— (1905b), On psychotherapy. *Standard Edition*, 7:257–270. London: Hogan Press, 1955.

———— (1909), *Notes on a case of obsessional neurosis. Standard Edition*, 10:153–250. London: Hogarth Press, 1955.

———— (1912), *Recommendations to physicians practising psycho-analysis. Standard Edition*, 12:109–120. London: Hogarth Press, 1955.

———— (1915), *Observations on transference love. Standard Edition*, 12:157–174. London: Hogarth Press, 1955

———— (1918), *From the history of an infantile neurosis. Standard Edition*, 17:3–22. London: Hogarth Press, 1955.

———— (1919), *The uncanny. Standard Edition*, 17:217–252. London: Hogarth Press, 1955.

———— (1920), *The psychogenesis of a case of homosexuality in a woman. Standard Edition*, 18:145–172. London: Hogarth Press, 1955.

———— (1921), Letter. Rare Books and Manuscript Library of Columbia University, New York. First published in *Body Politic*. Toronto, Canada, May 1977: p. 9.

———— (1985), *The Complete Letters of Sigmund Freud to Wilhelm Fleiss*, ed. and trans. J. Masson. Cambridge, MA: Harvard University Press.

Frank, K. (1997), The role of the analyst's inadvertent self-revelations. *Psychoanal. Dial.*, 7:281–314.

Frommer, M. S. (2000), Offending gender: Being and wanting in male same-sex desire. *Studies Gender & Sexuality* 1:191–206.

Frye, N. (1957), *Anatomy of Criticism*. Princeton, NJ: Princeton University Press.

Gabbard, G. (1996), *Love and Hate in the Analytic Setting*. New York: Jason Aronson.

———— and Lester, E. P. (1995), *Boundaries and Boundary Violations in Psychoanalysis*. Washington DC: American Psychiatric Press.

Gay, P. (1990), *Freud: A Life for Our Time*. New York: Norton.

Gerson, B. ed., (1996), The Therapist as a Person: Life Crises, Life Experiences, and Their Effects on Treatment. Hillsdale, NJ: The Analytic Press.

Gilligan, C. (1982), *In a Different Voice: Psychological Theory and Women's Development*. Cambridge, MA: Harvard University Press.

Gilman, S. (1988), The iconography of disease. In: *AIDS: Cultural Analysis/Cultural Activism*, ed. D. Crimp. Cambridge, MA: MIT Press, pp. 87– 107.

Goffman, E. (1963), *Stigma: Notes on the Management of Spoiled Identity*. New York: Simon & Schuster.

Gold, J. H. (1993), Introduction. In: *Beyond Transference: When the Therapist's Real*

Life Intrudes, ed. J. H. Gold & J. C. Nemiah. Washington, DC: American Psychiatric Press, pp. ix–xii.

Goldman, S. (1989), Bearing the unbearable. In: *Gender in Transition*, ed. J. Offerman Zuckerberg. New York: Plenum, pp. 263–274.

Goldstein, E. (1994), Self-Disclosure in treatment: What therapists do and don't talk about. *Clin. Soc. Work J.*, 22:417–434.

——— (1997), To tell or not to tell. *Clin. Soc. Work J.*, 25:41–58.

Greenberg, J. (1995), Self-disclosure: Is it psychoanalytic? *Contemp. Psychoanal.* 31:193–205.

Grosz, S. (1993), A phantasy of infection. *Internat. J. Psycho-Anal.*, 74:965–974.

Grotstein, J. (1994), "The old order changeth"—A reassessment of the basic rule of psychoanalytic technique. *Psychoanal. Dial.*, 4:595–608.

Grunbaum, A. (1984), *The Foundations of Psychoanalysis: A Philosophical Critique*. Berkeley, CA: University of California Press.

Halpert, E. (1982), When the analyst is chronically ill or dying. *Psychoanal. Quart.*, 51:372–389.

Hamer, D., & Copeland, P. (1994), *The Science of Desire: The Search for the Gay Gene And the Biology of Behavior*. New York: Simon & Schuster.

Harris, A. (1998), Psychic envelopes and sonorous baths: Siting the body in relational theory and clinical practice. In: *Relational Perspectives on the Body*, ed. L. Aron & F. Anderson. Hillsdale, NJ: The Analytic Press, pp. 39–64.

Hartmann, H. (1960), *Psychoanalysis and Moral Values*. New York: International Universities Press.

Hay, L. (1986), Self healing: Creating your health. Audiotape. Carlsbad, CA.: Hayhouse.

Heidegger, M. (1972), *On Time and Being*, tr. J. Stambaugh. New York: Harper & Row.

Heimann, P. (1950), On countertransference. *Internat. J. Psycho-Anal.*, 31:81–84.

Hildebrand, H. P. (1992), A patient dying with AIDS. *Internat. Rev. Psycho-Anal.*, 19:457–469.

Hindle, M. (1993), Introduction. *Dracula*, by B. Stoker. New York: Penguin.

Hoffer, A. (1985), Toward a definition of psychoanalytic neutrality. *J. Amer. Psychoanal. Assn.*, 33:771.

Hoffman, I. (1998), *Ritual and Spontaneity in the Psychoanalytic Process*. Hillsdale, NJ: The Analytic Press.

Iasenza, S. & Glassgold, J. (1995), *Lesbians and Psychoanalysis*. New York: Free Press.

Isay, R. (1989), *Being Homosexual*. New York: Farrar, Straus & Giroux.

——— (1996), *Becoming Gay*. New York; Pantheon.

Jacobs, T. (1995), Discussion of Jay Greenberg's Paper. *Contemp. Psychoanal.*, 31:237–245.

Jones, E. (1957), *The Life and Work of Sigmund Freud, vol. III*. New York: Basic Books.

Johnson, D. (1991), Introduction. *Frankenstein*, by M. Shelley. New York: Bantam Books.

Kant, E. (1781) tr. N. K. Smith. *Critique of Pure Reason*. New York: St. Martin's, 1965.

——— (1785) tr. J. Ellington. *Grounding for the Metaphysics of Morals*. Indianapolis: Hackett, 1993.

Kappraff, A. (1995), Boundaries of time and space in the treatment of HIV-positive man in mid-life. *Bull. Menn. Clin.*, 59:69–78.

Kaufmann, W. (1968), *Nietzsche*. Princeton, NJ: Princeton University Press.

Kernberg, O. (1965), Notes on countertransference. *J. Amer. Psychoanal. Assn.*, 13:38–56.

Klein, M. (1957), *Envy and Gratitude and Other Works*. London: Tavistock.

Kobayashi, J. S. (1997), The evolution of adjustment issues in HIV/AIDS. *Bull. Menn. Clin.*, 61:146–188.

Kohut, H. (1971), *The Analysis of the Self.* Madison, CT: International Universities Press.

——— (1984), *How Does Analysis Cure?* ed. A. Goldberg & Paul Stepansky. Chicago: University of Chicago Press.

Kraemer, S. (1996), "Betwixt the dark and the daylight" of maternal subjectivity: Meditations on the threshold. *Psychoanal. Dial.*, 6:765–791.

Lacan, J. (1977), *Ecrits*. New York: Norton.

Laplanche, J. & Pontalis, J. B.(1983), *The Language of Psychoanalysis*. London: Hogarth Press.

Lasky, R. (1990), Catastrophic illness in the analyst and the analyst's emotional reactions to it. *Internat. J. Psycho-Anal.*, 71:455–473.

——— (1992), Some superego conflicts in the analyst who has suffered a catastrophic illness. *Internat. J. Psycho-Anal.*, 73:127–136.

Lazar, S. (1990), Patient's responses to pregnancy and miscarriage in the analyst. In: *Illness in the Analyst: Implications for the Treatment Relationship*, ed. H. J. Schwartz & A. S. Silver. Madison, CT: International Universities Press, pp. 199–226.

Leary, K. (1994), Psychoanalytic "problems" and postmodern "solutions". *Psychoanal. Quart.*, 63:433–465.

Lehrer, R. (1995), *Nietzsche's Presence in Freud's Life and Work*. Albany: State University of New York Press.

Levy-Suhl, M. (1946), The role of ethics and religion in psycho-analytic theory and therapy. *Internat. J. Psycho-Anal.*, 27:110–119.

Lewes, K. (1988), *The Psychoanalytic Theory of Male Homosexuality*. New York: Simon & Schuster.

Linton, S. (1998), *Claiming Disability: Knowledge and Identity*. New York: New York University Press.

Lopate, P. (1995), *The Art of the Personal Essay*. New York: Anchor Books.

Lorde, A. (1982), *Zamie: A New Spelling of My Name*. New York: Crossing.

Magee, M. & Miller, D. (1999), *Lesbian Lives: Psychoanalytic Narratives Old and New*. Hillsdale, NJ: The Analytic Press.

Mass, L. (1994), *Confessions of a Jewish Wagnerite*. New York: Cassel.

Masson, J. M. (1985), *The Complete Letters of Sigmund Freud to Wilhelm Fleiss, 1887–1904*. Cambridge, MA: Harvard University Press.

Mayer, E. L. (1994), Some implications for psychoanalytic technique drawn from the analysis of a dying patient. *Psychoanal. Quart.*, 63:1–19.

Mayers, A. M. & Svartberg, M. (1996), The manifestation and management of countertransference on a pediatric AIDS team. *Bull. Menn. Clin.*, 60:206–218.

McLaughlin, J. (1961), The analyst and the Hippocratic Oath. *J. Amer. Psychoanal. Assn.*, 9:106–123.

Meissner, W. (1994), Psychoanalysis and ethics: Beyond the pleasure principle. *Contemp. Psychoanal.*, 30:453–472.

Mendelsohn, D. (1999), *The Elusive Embrace: Desire and the Riddle of Identity.* New York: Knopf.

Michaels, J. (1969), Guides on professional conduct for psychoanalysts. *J. Amer. Psychoanal. Assn.*, 17:291–311.

Mileno, M., Barnowski, C., Fiore, T., Gormley, J., Rich, J., Emgushov, R-T., & Carpenter, C. (2001), Factitious HIV syndrome in young women. *The AIDS Reader*, 11:263–268.

Miller, D. A. (1992), *Bringing Out Roland Barthes.* Berkeley: University of California Press.

Mitchell, J. (1982), Introduction. *Feminine Sexuality* by J. Lacan, ed. J. Mitchell & J. Rose. New York: Norton.

Mitchell, S. (1988a), *Relational Concepts in Psychoanalysis: An Integration.* Cambridge MA: Harvard University Press.

——— (1988b), Clinical implications of the developmental tilt. In: *Relational Concepts in Psychoanalysis: An Integration.* Cambridge MA: Harvard University Press, pp. 151–172.

——— (1993), *Hope and Dread in Psychoanalysis.* New York: Basic Books.

Money-Kyrle, R. (1952), Psycho-analysis and ethics. *Internat. J. Psycho-Anal.*, 33:225–234.

Monette, P. (1988), *Borrowed Time: An AIDS Memoir.* New York: Harcourt Brace Jovanovich.

Moore, B. E. & Fine, B. D. eds. (1990), *Psychoanalytic Terms and Concepts.* New Haven, CT: Yale University Press.

Morrison, A. L. (1990), Doing psychotherapy while living with a life-threatening illness. In *Illness and the Analyst: Implications for treatment*, ed. H. Schwartz and A. L. Silver. Madison, CT: International Universities Press, pp. 227–252.

——— (1997), Ten years of doing psychotherapy while living with a life threatening illness: Self-disclosure and other ramifications. *Psychoanal. Dial.*, 7:225–242.

Moustakas, C. (1990), *Heuristic Research: Design, Methodology and Applications.* Newbury Park, CA: Sage.

Nagle, T. (1986), *The View From Nowhere.* Oxford: Oxford University Press.

National Association of Social Workers (1996), Code of Ethics. Washington, DC: National Association of Social Workers.

Nielson, N. (1960), Value judgements in psychoanalysis. *Internat. J. Psycho-Anal.* 41:425–429.

Nietzsche, F. (1887) tr. W. Kaufman. *On the Genealogy of Morals.* New York: Vintage Books, 1989.

O'Connor, N. & Ryan, J. (1993), *Wild Desires and Mistaken Identities.* New York: Columbia University Press.

Odets, W. (1995), *In the Shadow of the Epidemic.* Durham, NC: Duke University Press.

Olsson, P. A. (1997), Time compressed: Psychoanalysis in the days of HIV and AIDS. *J. Amer. Acad. Psychoanal.*, 25:277–293.

Orange, D. (1995), *Emotional Understanding: Studies in Psychoanalytic Epistemology.* New York: Guilford Press.

Pizer, B. (2000), The therapist's routine consultations: A necessary window in the treatment frame. *Psychoanal. Dial.*, 10:197–208.

Pizer, S. (1998), *Building Bridges: The Negotiation of Paradox in Psychoanalysis.* Hillsdale, NJ: The Analytic Press.

Pleck, J. H. (1995), The gender role strain paradigm: An update. In: *A New Psychology of Men*, ed. R. F. Levant & W. S. Pollack. New York: Basic Books, pp. 11–32..

Plato (n. d.) *The Complete Texts of Great Dialogues of Plato*, tr. W. H. D. Rouse. New York: Plume, 1970.

Poe, E. A. (1845), *The Fall of the House of Usher and Other Writings.* New York: Penguin, 1986.

Racker, H. (1957), The meanings and uses of countertransference. *Psychoanal. Quart.*, 26:303–357.

——— (1966), Ethics and psycho-analysis and the psycho-analysis of ethics. *Internat. J. Psycho-Anal.*, 47:63–80.

Renik, O. (1993), Analytic interaction: Conceptualizing technique in the light of the analyst's irreducible subjectivity. *Psychoanal. Quart.*, 62:553–571.

——— (1995a), The role of an analyst's expectations in clinical technique: Reflections on the concept of resistance *J. Amer. Psychoanal. Assn.*, 43:83–94.

——— (1995b), The ideal of the anonymous analyst and the problem of self-disclosure. *Psychoanal. Quart.*, 64:466–495.

——— (1999), Playing one's cards face up in analysis: An approach to the problem of self disclosure. *Psychoanal. Quart.*, 68:521–540.

Reich, A. (1951), On countertransference. *Internat. J. Psycho-Anal.*, 32:25–31.

——— (1960), Further remarks on countertransference. *Internat. J. Psycho-Anal.*, 41:389–395.

Ricoeur, P. (1984), *Time and Narrative Vol. 1.* Chicago: University of Chicago Press.

——— (1992), *Oneself as Another.* Chicago: University of Chicago Press.

Rofes, E. (1998), *Dry Bones Breathe: Gay Men Creating Post-AIDS Identities.* New York: Harrington Park Press.

Rosenbaum, M. (1994), Similarities of psychiatric disorders of AIDS and syphilis: History repeats itself. *Bull. Menn. Clin.*, 58:375–382.

Sadowy, D. (1991), Is there a role for the psychoanalytic psychotherapist with a patient dying of AIDS? *Psychoanal. Rev.*, 78:199–207.

Scarce, M. (1999), A ride on the wild side. *POZ Magazine*, February, 1999: p. 52.

Schafer, R. (1983), *The Analytic Attitude.* New York: Basic Books.

Schaffner, B. (1994), The crucial and difficult role of the psychotherapist in the treatment of the HIV-positive patient. *J. Amer. Acad. Psychoanal.*, 22:505–518.

——— (1997), Modifying psychoanalytic methods when treating the HIV-positive patient. *J. Amer. Acad. Psychoanal.*, 25:123–141.

Scheffler, S. (1992), *Human Morality.* New York: Oxford Press.

Schoenberg, E. & Lesser, R. (eds.) (1999), *That Obscure Object of Desire: Freud's Female Homosexual Revisited.* New York: Routledge.

Schwartz, A. (1998), *Sexual Subjects: Lesbians, Gender, and Psychoanalysis.* New York: Routledge.

Schwartz, H. J. (1987), Illness in the doctor: Implications for the psychoanalytic process. *J. Amer. Psychoanal. Assn.*, 35: 657–692.

——— & Silver, A. L. S. eds. (1990), *Illness in the Analyst: Implications for the Treatment Relationship.* Madison, CT: International Universities Press.

Schwartzberg, S. (1993), Struggling for meaning: How HIV-positive gay men make sense of AIDS. *Profess. Psychol.: Research & Practice*, 24:483–490.

——— (1994), Vitality and growth in HIV-infected gay men. *Soc. Sci. Med.*, 38:593–602.

Serota, H. (1976), Ethics, moral values and psychological interventions. *Internat. J. Psycho-Anal.*, 3:373–375.

Shelley, M. (1816), *Frankenstein, or the Modern Prometheus.* New York: Bantam Books, 1991.

Shernoff, M. (1991), Eight years of working with people with HIV: The impact upon a therapist. In *Gays, Lesbians, and their Therapists*, ed. C. Silverstein. New York: Norton, pp. 227–239.

——— (1996), The last journey: Remaining fully alive in the face of death (psychotherapy with people with AIDS). *Family Therapy Networker*, Jan.–Feb.

Silver, A. (1982), Resuming the work with a life-threatening illness. *Contemp. Psychoanal.* 18:314–326.

Simon, W. (1996), *Postmodern Sexualities.* New York: Routledge.

Socarides, C. (1968), *Homosexuality.* Northvale, NJ: Jason Aronson.

Sontag, S. (1988), *AIDS and its Metaphors.* New York: Farrar, Straus & Giroux.

Spence, D. P. (1987), *The Freudian Metaphor: Toward Paradigm Change in Psychoanalysis.* New York: Norton.

Stade, G. (1981), Introduction. *Dracula* by B. Stoker. New York: Bantam Classics.

Stanislavsky, C. (1989), *An Actor Prepares.* New York: Theatre Arts Books.

Stark, M. (1951), *Child of Light: A Reassessment of Mary Wollstonecraft Shelley.* Hadleigh, Essex, UK: Tower Bridge.

Steiner, W. (1999), Introduction. *Frankenstein* by M. Shelley. New York: Modern Library.

Stepansky, P. (1999), *Freud, Surgery, and the Surgeons.* Hillsdale, NJ: The Analytic Press.

Stern, D. (1985), *The Interpersonal World of the Infant.* New York: Basic Books.

Stern, D. B. (1997), *Unformulated Experience: From Dissociation to Imagination in Psychoanalysis.* Hillsdale, NJ: The Analytic Press.

Stevens, I. A. & Muskin, P. R. (1987), Techniques for reversing the failure of empathy towards AIDS patients. *J. Amer. Acad. Psychoanal.*, 15:539–552.

Stoker, B. (1897), *Dracula.* New York: Bantam Classics, 1981.

Stone, L. (1961), *Transference and its Context.* New York: Aronson.

Taylor, M. (1987), *Altarity.* Chicago: University of Chicago Press.

Teicholz, J. (1999), *Kohut, Loewald, and the Postmoderns: A Comparative Study of Self and Relationship*. Hillsdale, NJ: The Analytic Press.

Treichler, R. (1988), AIDS, homophobia, and biomedical discourse: An epidemic of signification. In *AIDS: Cultural Analysis/Cultural Activism*, ed. D. Crimp. Cambridge, MA: MIT Press. pp. 31–70.

Wallerstein, R. (1976), Introduction to symposium on "Ethics, Moral Values and Psychological Interventions." *Internat. Rev. Psycho-Anal.*, 3:369–372.

Warner, M. (1999), *The Trouble with Normal: Sex, Politics, and the Ethics of Queer Life*. New York: Free Press.

Watney, S. (1988), The spectacle of AIDS. In: *AIDS: Cultural Analysis/Cultural Activism*, ed. D.Crimp. Cambridge, MA: MIT Press. pp. 71–86.

White, E. (1994), *The Burning Library: Essays*. New York: Vintage.

White, H.(1990), *The Content of the Form: Narrative Discourse and Historical Representation*. Baltimore: Johns Hopkins University Press.

Winnicott, D. W. (1951), Transitional objects and transitional phenomena. In *Playing and Reality*. London: Tavistock, 1971, pp. 1–25.

——— (1960), Ego distortion in terms of true and false self. In *The Maturational Processes and the Facilitating Environment*. Madison, CT: International Universities Press, 1965, pp. 140–152.

——— (1969), The use of an object and relating through identifications. In *Playing and Reality*. London: Tavistock, 1971, pp. 88–94.

Wolf, L. (1992), Introduction. *Dracula* by Bram Stoker. New York: Signet Classic

Wong, N. (1990), Acute illness in the analyst. In: *Illness in the Analyst: Implications for the Treatment Relationship*. Ed. H. J. Schwartz & A. L. S. Silver. Madison, CT: International Universities Press, pp. 27–46.

INDEX